THE
FAMILY
GOOD HEALTH GUIDE

THE
FAMILY
GOOD HEALTH GUIDE
Common Sense on Common Health Problems
By
Dr John Fry
Dr Alistair Moulds
Dr Gillian Strube Dr Eric Gambrill

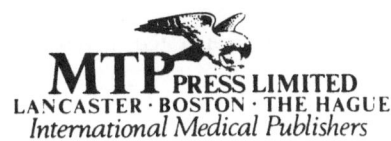

MTP PRESS LIMITED
LANCASTER · BOSTON · THE HAGUE
International Medical Publishers

Published in the UK and Europe by
MTP Press Limited
Falcon House
Lancaster, England

British Library Cataloguing in Publication Data

The Family good health guide.
  1. Health
  I. Fry, John
  613   RA776

    ISBN-13: 978-94-011-6245-6   e-ISBN-13: 978-94-011-6243-2
    DOI: 10.1007/978-94-011-6243-2

Published in the USA by
MTP Press
A division of Kluwer Boston Inc
190 Old Derby Street
Hingham, MA 02043, USA

Phototypeset by Swiftpages Limited, Liverpool, Merseyside

Contents

Preface

Although we have no good definition of 'health', all people have their own ideas of whether they are healthy or not. Based on personal experience and knowledge each person comes to accept that within themselves there is a normal range of feelings and performance, departure from which could be considered abnormal or unhealthy.

Despite the many amazing technological advances made over recent decades it cannot be said that access to advanced medical care is the main determining factor in the healthiness or otherwise of a society. Even in these modern times most diseases and health problems are non-curable in the strict sense, and the scope for effective prevention of disease is more limited than some enthusiasts suggest.

Individuals must appreciate the limitations of modern medical care and, while seeking to use the care available to best possible effect, accept that the responsibility for trying to prevent major disease rests in their own hands.

In this book we have tried to present a balanced and realistic picture of the many factors that must be taken into account if optimum disease prevention and health maintenance are to be achieved. The health of your family is your responsibility. An understanding of what can go wrong, how it can be prevented or how it can best be coped with can only be helpful to you.

PART I

1
Health and non-health

One half of married life is directly concerned with bringing up our children. As each generation of parents undertakes this task they come to face the common and well-nigh inevitable problems.

Despite the fact that mortality in childhood and in young adults has fallen dramatically and that major 'old diseases' such as tuberculosis, poliomyelitis, pneumonia, rheumatic fever, and the effects of inadequate food, warmth, and shelter have been controlled, there is no reduction in the total incidence of illness that exists in our modern society (Figures 1.1 and 1.2). Figure 1.1 shows the continuing decrease in mortality in the UK over the past 140 years with the rate being always higher in men. Figure 1.2 is a composite approximation of 'morbidity', shown as the rate of use of family-physician services, use of drugs, hospitalization, and sickness-insurance demands have increased. This 'morbidity rate' has increased; and the rate for women has always been higher.

With many more physicians and nurses at work more busily than ever before and with more and more hospitals admitting and caring for more and more people there is no evidence that we are curing, preventing, or wiping out disease (Figures 1.3 and 1.4). It is as though there is a *vacuum of sophistication*; even as we have controlled tuberculosis, pneumonia, poliomyelitis, etc., so into the vacuum have rushed other, less major disorders.

We are living longer than before; but are we living better? The life

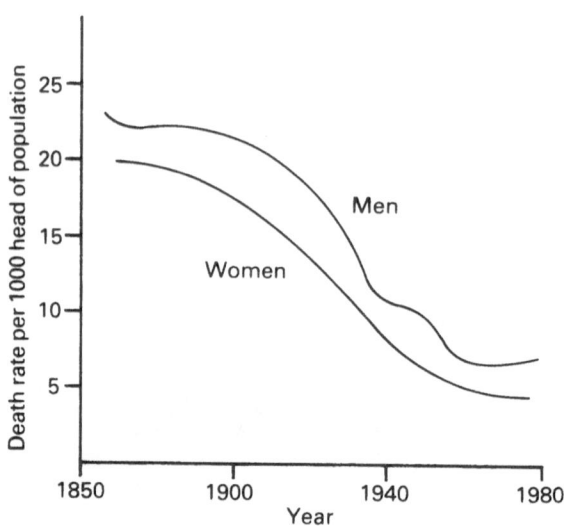

Figure 1.1   Death rate per 1000 head of population, 1850—1980.

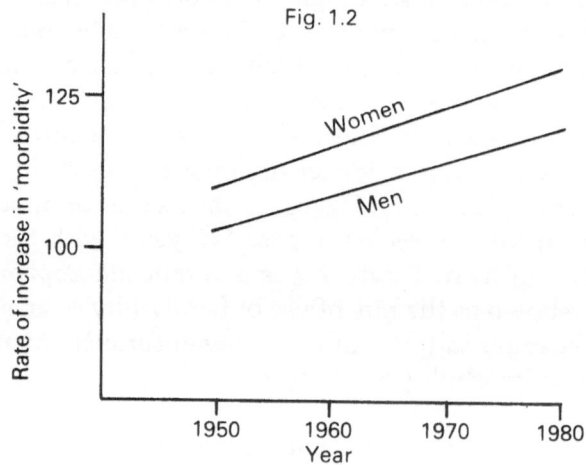

Figure 1.2   Rate of increase in morbidity, 1950—1980.

expectancy of a male now is around 73 years and of a female 76 years. However, when the reasons for our expectations to live beyond three score and ten years are examined, they show that it is because of safer childbirth and fewer deaths in infancy that we are living longer. Fifty years ago it was not unusual in Europe and North America for up to one child in five not to live beyond the first year (Figure 1.5).

The life expectancy of a man aged 40 now has increased by only 4 — 5 years above that of his grandfather at the same age half a century ago. The reason for this is that we have not improved our health all that much from middle age onwards, and this is probably related directly to bad health habits that we develop as young men and women.

The incidence of personal physical, mental, and social illness appears to be increasing. One indication of this is that children suffer from just as much if not more illness; there is a much greater tendency for persons to suffer from mental—emotional disorders; there is much

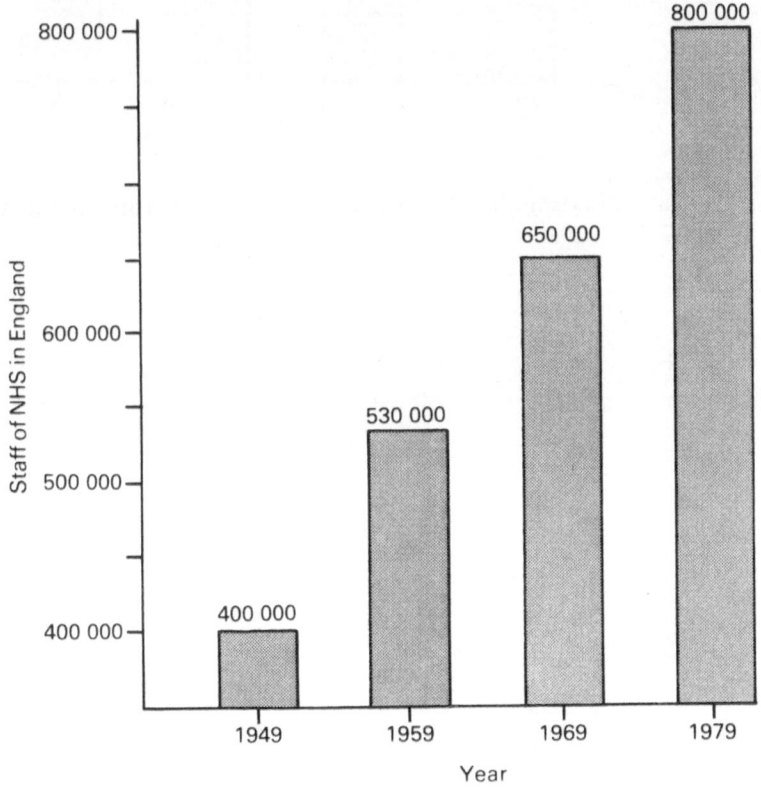

Figure 1.3 Numbers of staff in NHS in England, 1949—1979.

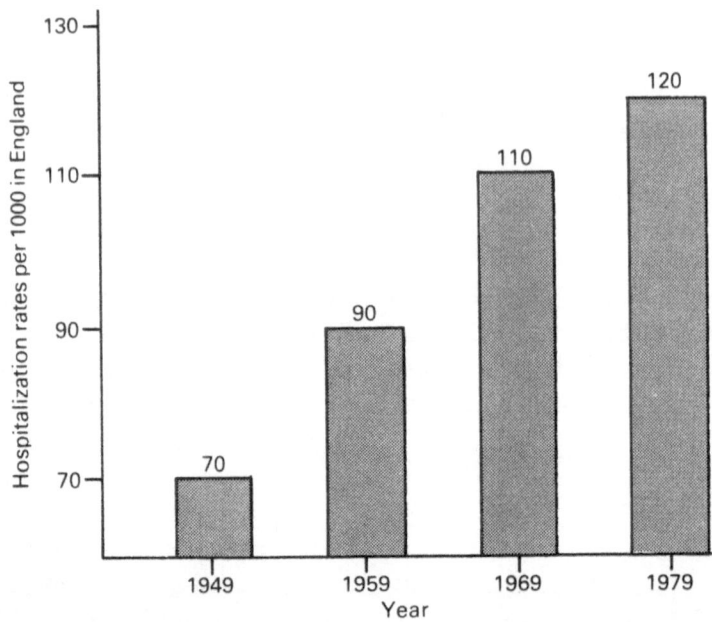

Figure 1.4   Rates of hospitalization per 1000 head of population in England, 1949–1979.

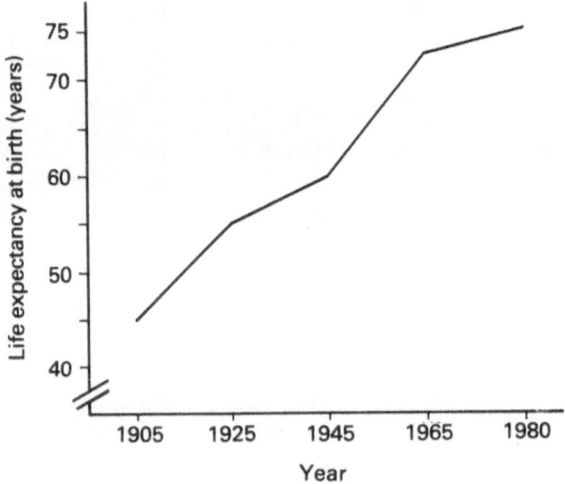

Figure 1.5   Life expectancy at birth in UK and USA, 1905–1980.

more family unhappiness and breakdown, as shown by increasing divorce rates; and there is much more social disorder, with crime and violence on the increase everywhere.

The young family

With these uncertainties in a less than perfect world, focusing attention on the young family offers the best hopes for a better future. It is in childhood and in young adult life that the foundations are laid down for a happy and a healthy future.

Young parents should acquire good habits that produce the ingredients for a healthy future, with attention to food, exercise, avoidance of smoking and excessive eating and drinking; to creating regular routines and self-discipline; and to developing a sound and common-sense philosophy for personal and family life.

It is also important that parents accept responsibilities to transmit sound principles for a good and healthy life to their children. Above all, they should teach them to accept personal responsibilities to attain and maintain good health and on how to prevent and avoid disease and accidents.

Modern problems and difficulties

Yet, despite the world in which we live — filled with modern techno-logical advances that have added to life's material comforts — young families have major problems to face.

The world is less secure and less stable. Economic disorder abounds; inflation is rampant; it is difficult to get started with house purchasing, and difficult to achieve personal ambitions and standards. Marriages are unstable, with 1 in 3 ending in divorce. The basis of marriage is being questioned, and many couples with children live together without solemnizing marriage. The number of single-parent families is increasing and so are the numbers of social orphans; children whose parents have deserted them. Family kinship is weaker and the extended family is less evident. With smaller family size and with a more-mobile society, there is less support from around-the-corner parents, grand-parents, uncles and aunts, and brothers and sisters. Young families are on their own much more — often in new and unfamiliar anonymous urban surroundings — and have to rely increasingly on uncertain friends and neighbours and on impersonal social services rather than on their own family roots and ties. The status of women and wives has changed. Many wives and mothers work, and try to be successful both as part-time mothers and part-time salaried workers.

These social upheavals and changes have created smaller and more-isolated and independent families. Young parents are better educated and better informed than ever before and are ambitious, expectant, and demanding of a good life. With one or two wanted and precious children there is constant striving for perfection and desire to do the very best for one's children to make their future even better and easier.

It comes as a shock when reality-gaps appear: when life and health become less than perfect; when set expectations cannot be met; when fond but impossible ambitions must be jettisoned; and when the reality dawns that we must live with the possible. Life becomes easier when an equilibrium between the possible and the common-sensical can be developed; this is the principal message of this book.

What is health?

Surprisingly, there is no good definition of 'health'. The World Health Organization (WHO) has one: 'a state of complete physical, mental and social well-being, and not merely an absence of disease' — but this is a Utopian ideal that is transient and eludes most of us for most of the time. There is no clear black-and-white distinction between health and non-health. There is a spectrum (Figure 1.6) ranging from health to sickness. At any time, fewer than 10% of us are 'healthy' by WHO standards and most are in a vague state of fair and sub-health, with probably only 20% under active medical care.

To put this another way, Figure 1.7 shows the proportions of persons who at any time are healthy, those who are self-caring for health problems, those who are receiving care from their personal physicians, and those who are being treated at hospital.

What is normal?

Another difficulty is to decide on what is 'normal'? As for 'health', a definition is scarcely possible. Better to accept that within ourselves we come to know a normal range of feelings and performance and that departure from these is 'abnormal'.

On a wider and less personal level there are certain 'abnormal' feelings, symptoms, or ailments that are so common and inevitable

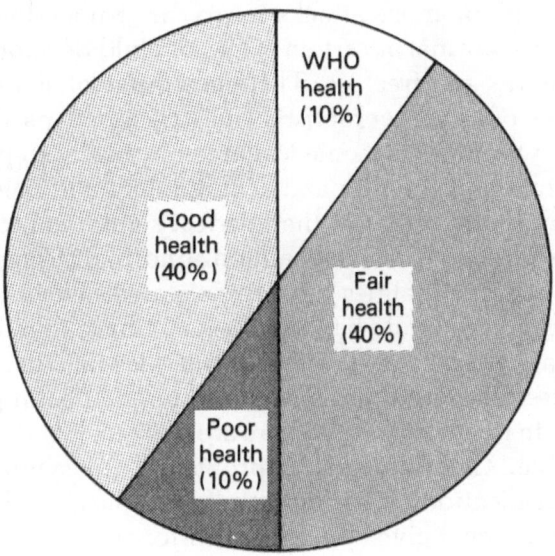

Figure 1.6 States of health of UK population.

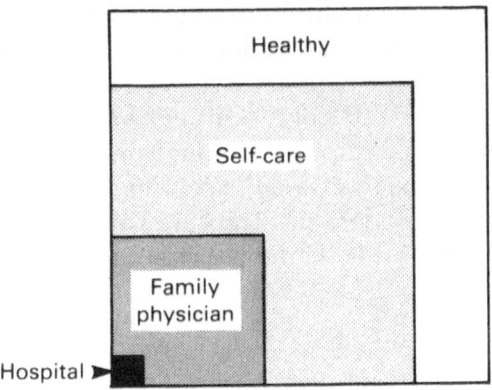

Figure 1.7 Proportions of UK population who are healthy, or receiving various degrees of treatment for health problems.

that they have to be accepted as 'normal abnormalities'. As examples there are the swings of mood from elation to depression that affect us all and influence our behaviour and temperament within ourselves and towards others. The common cold and its variants — with nasal discharge, obstruction, and cough — are well-nigh inevitable and each of us suffers one or more attacks in a year. Knock-knees and bow (bandy) legs are normal at certain stages of child development, as are many birthmarks and freckles. There is a range of statistical normal weight but few of us are ever satisfied with their own particular weight or shape. As we age we become less able physically to perform tasks easily undertaken in the past and aching joints and muscles become accepted as normal, as do less than perfect sight and hearing.

The final arbiter on what is a common abnormality may have to be a physician. But some realities have to be stated. The old saying that medical endeavours should be: 'to cure sometimes, to relieve often, to comfort always — and to prevent hopefully' is still true.

Even in these modern times most diseases and health problems are *non-curable*, in the strict sense. There are few quick and ready specific cures available. Certainly, many problems and symptoms can be *relieved* by medication or through medical or surgical therapies. The art of good care, be it given by the professional nurse or physician or by a parent or friend, must be to 'comfort always'. Support, reassurance, and optimism are an essential ingredient of caring. The scope for effective *prevention* is more limited than some enthusiasts suggest. The benefits of immunization for a few infective diseases is acknowledged but medical screening and check-up are of doubtful benefit. The prevention of some major modern diseases such as some cancers, heart disease, and stroke is through better self-care and health maintenance; through avoiding smoking, over-eating and drinking; and through regular exercise and life routine.

The limitations of modern medical care have to be accepted; some problems and symptoms have to be tolerated and lived with.

Common diseases

'Common diseases are those that occur commonly and rare diseases are those that rarely happen.

Figure 1.8 shows the relative proportions of the common diseases of

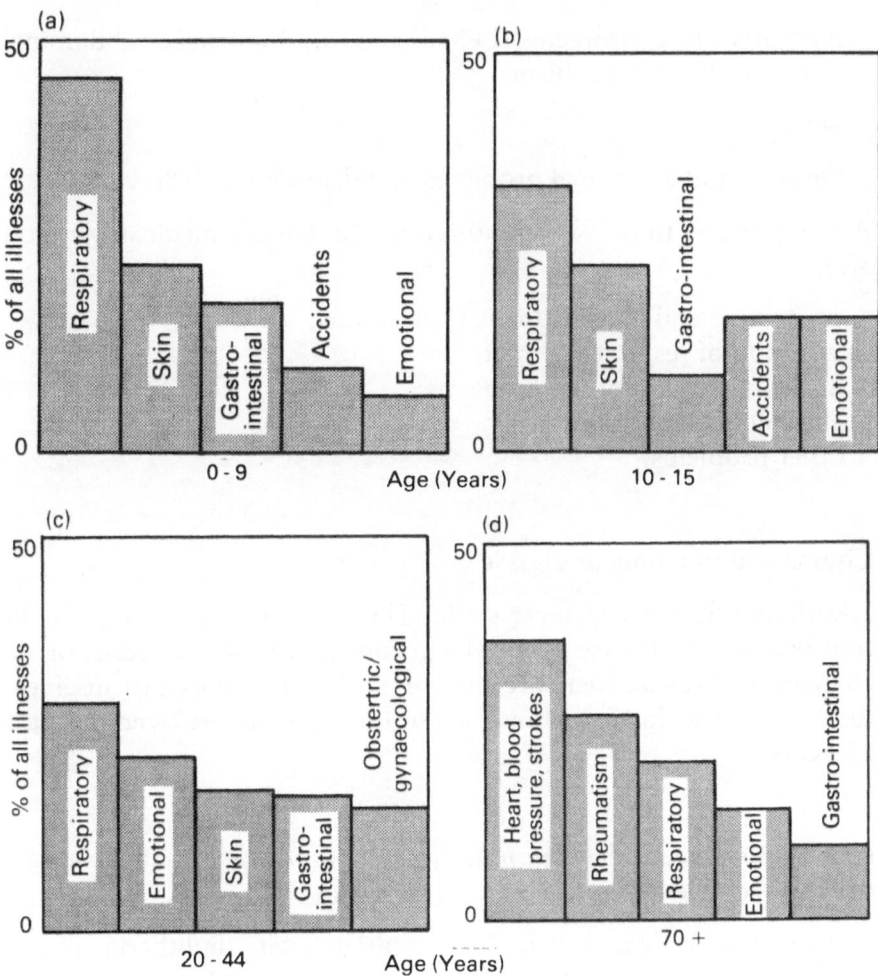

Figure 1.8 Relative proportions of common diseases in: (a) and (b) childhood; (c) parents; (d) grandparents.

childhood (0—9 and 10—15 years) and those of parents (25—44 years)
and grandparents (aged 70 and over). Taking *childhood* as a whole the
most common reasons for seeking medical attention are, in order:

infections of the respiratory tract, i.e. coughs, colds, earaches, sore
throats and bronchitis;

skin disorders;

gastrointestinal problems, i.e. sickness and diarrhoea, abdominal pains, and eating problems;

accidents;

nervous and emotional problems and disorders of behaviour.

Among *parents* the most common causes for seeking medical attention are:

pregnancy and gynaecological conditions;
infection of respiratory tract;
nervous and emotional problems;
gastrointestinal disorders;
other problems.

Course and outcome of disease

Health and disease are never static. There are constant changes over time because the diseases themselves change, because the quality of life changes, or because there are changes within individuals themselves. Recent medical history shows some ups and downs over the past 25 years.

Diseases which have become much less common or more controlled by medical treatment

Infections — such as tuberculosis, scarlet fever, diphtheria, polio-myelitis, whooping cough, tetanus, pneumonia, and skin infections. This is because of immunization and antibiotics.

Ulcers of the stomach and duodenum, because of safer surgery and more effective drugs.
High blood pressure, because of more effective drugs.
Asthma, because of more effective drugs.
Depression and other mental disorders, because of more effective drugs.

Safer childbirth and care of infants, because of better understanding and improved methods.

Diseases which have become more common

Coronary-artery diseases and heart failure.
Lung cancer.
Strokes.
Alcoholism.
Accidents.
Rheumatism and arthritis.

Time dimensions

The time dimension in disease shows five patterns (Figure 1.9).

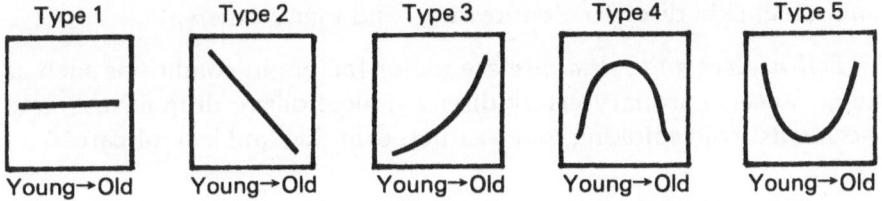

Figure 1.9   The five types of patterns that a disease can take (see text).

Type 1 is conditions that, once present, remain *unchanged for the remainder of life*, i.e. certain birth deformities, paralysis, and diabetes.

Type 2 is disorders of childhood which *children tend to outgrow*, such as coughs, colds, earaches, sore throats, wheezy chests, tummy aches, knock-knees and bow legs, and birth marks and bulging navels.

Type 3 is *disorders of ageing* that become more common and more severe with age (after 50), i.e. cancers, heart disease, bronchitis, rheumatism, strokes, and high blood pressure.

Type 4 is the pattern of some diseases that start in early adult life, persist for some 5–10 years and then *cease spontaneously*, i.e. duo-denal ulcers, hay fevers, lumbago, cystitis, asthma, migraine, and some depressions.

Type 5 is disorders that appear *most often in childhood and in the elderly*, i.e. hernia, constipation, and some others.

Causes and treatment

Our understanding of the nature and causes of common diseases is limited. Broadly, the causes can be put as follows:

External agents such as infecting micro-organisms like bacteria and viruses; pollutants of, and additives in, foods, water, and air; radio-activity; and the varied stresses and strains of life.

Possible known causes of conditions such as coronary-artery diseases, high blood pressure, strokes, and some cancers — but knowledge about these possibilities is far from clear or complete.

Unknown causes of conditions such as rheumatism, stomach ulcers; migraine, skin disorders, depression, and many others.

Self-neglect and self-abuse are major factors in conditions such as lung cancer; coronary-artery diseases; alcoholism; drug misuse; and accidents from smoking, over-eating, drinking and lack of care.

Good health care

This must be an act of collaboration and co-operation between patients and doctors. Individuals and their families must try to understand the rules of health, health maintenance, disease prevention, and how best to use available health services.

Physicians must acknowledge that they are but members of a team providing care and preventing disease. Collaboration with others such as nurses, social workers, and individual patients makes for success.

2
Family planning

There are now more than four billion people. An extra 70 million are born each year, and the population will go on doubling every 37 years or so (Table 2.1). Although the rate of increase is slowing, especially in the developed world, no amount of family planning can alter the number of people already here and the problems of pollution and the use of non-renewable natural resources, which are with us now, will continue to grow unless there is a determined effort to halt the growth.

Table 2.1   Years to double population in different world regions

Region	Years
World	37
Africa	26
Latin America	26
East Asia	42
South Asia	26
Indian subcontinent	30
Europe	115
North America	77
USSR	70
Australasia	35

In *developed countries* such as the USA and Britain nearly all women have access to modern contraception and each woman is likely to produce 1 or 2 children. Medical and social factors have lowered the infant death rate so that nearly all these babies are guaranteed a long life of three score years and ten.

In *developing countries* there is a very different pattern. A woman in the Third World will have 5 or 6 children during her life; 2 or 3 are likely to die in infancy. Three-quarters of the world population live in less-developed countries, where resources and technology are insufficient to control population growth.

However, most people do not think in global terms when planning their own families! They think more in terms of how many children they want, when they want to have them and, also, of what are the safest and most reliable methods of contraception available with which to achieve their objectives.

Current methods undoubtedly allow couples to exercise a very high degree of control over their own reproduction and help to ensure that no unwanted, unwelcomed, or unloved baby need be born (Table 2.2).

Table 2.2   Estimated percentage of couples using birth control*

Method	Percentage (world-wide)
Sterilization	28
Pill	19
Sheath	12
Coil	5
Abortion	14
Withdrawal, rhythm, and others	22

*It is estimated that over 290 million couples in the world are using some form of birth control.

In Britain and the USA the *pill* is the most popular method of birth control, especially among younger women — although its popularity wanes with increased age. In more than one in three couples who have completed their families, one or other partner has been *sterilized*. The *diaphragm* (cap) is becoming more popular in the USA, while the *sheath* retains its popularity in Britain. In both countries about 8% of women requiring contraception are fitted with a *coil* (IUD). As an indicator of contraceptive failure, it must be noted that 30% of pregnancies in the USA and 14% in Britain are ended by *legally induced abortion*.

Structure and function

Female cycle

Shortly after puberty (at about 13 years of age), hormone changes in the developing body trigger off the first discharge of the blood and tissue lining of the womb. This process is known as *menstruation* and it recurs approximately every 4 weeks until it finally stops at the *menopause*, which takes place when the woman is aged about 50 years.

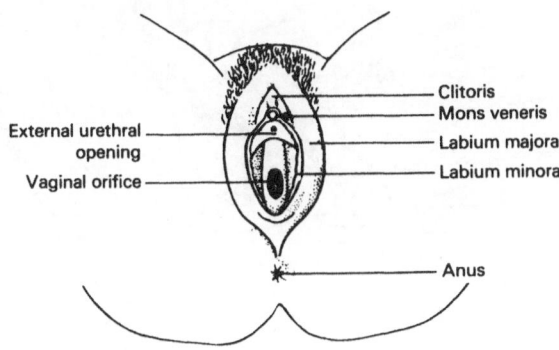

Figure 2.1   Female sex organs, external view.

At the beginning of each cycle the egg (ovum) develops in the ovary and the hormone, oestrogen, is produced. On about the fourteenth day the egg is released from the ovary and starts to travel down the Fallopian tube to the womb (uterus). The ovary also makes the other sex hormone, which is called progesterone, and under the influence of this and oestrogen the lining of the womb becomes thicker.

If a sperm manages to travel up through the womb and into the Fallopian tube at the time the egg is released then it will fuse with the egg, so fertilizing it. The fertilized egg will then travel to embed itself in the womb lining, with the egg then developing into the baby, and the womb lining developing into the placenta (afterbirth).

When fertilization does not occur the egg dies (it lives for

24—48 hours only), and in 14 days hormone production from the ovary stops and causes the womb lining to be cast off. This produces the 3—4 ounces of blood during menstruation and after it is passed a new cycle will begin.

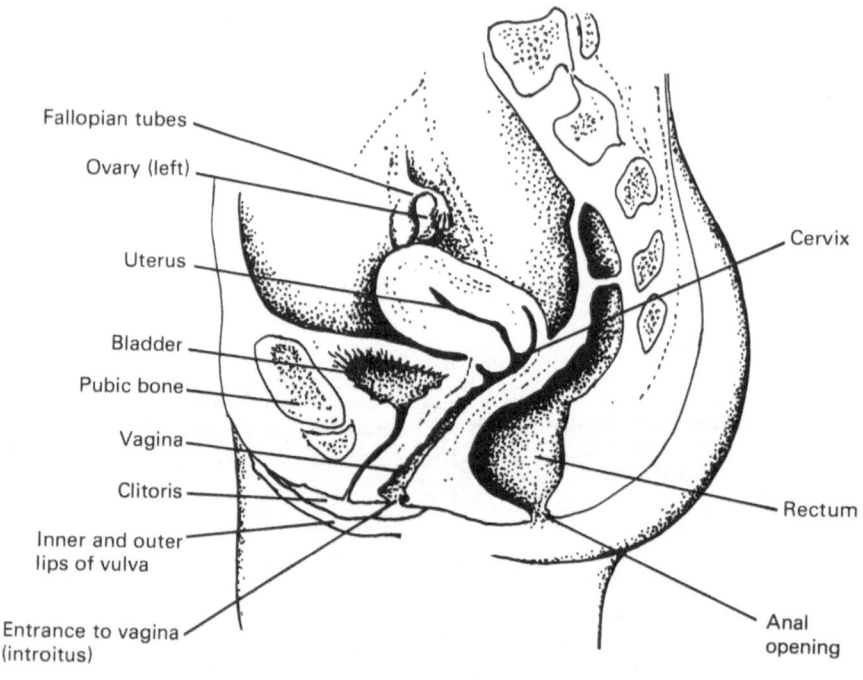

Fallopian tubes

Ovary (left)

Uterus

Bladder

Pubic bone

Vagina

Clitoris

Inner and outer lips of vulva

Entrance to vagina (introitus)

Cervix

Rectum

Anal opening

Figure 2.2 Section through midline of female pelvis (female genital tract seen from the side).

Male function

Sperms are continuously produced in the testicles and move up the vas deferens to be stored until released in seminal fluid during ejaculation. Nearly 200 million are released each time. In male sterilization (vasectomy) small incisions are made on each side of the scrotum with division of the vas. Sperms can no longer go up the vas and once those that are in store have been used up the man becomes sterile. This clearing of the tubes occurs after about 20 ejaculations and affects only the sperms. The fluid in which they were stored is still produced and so even after vasectomy, the sex act — with ejaculation and orgasm — is unaltered.

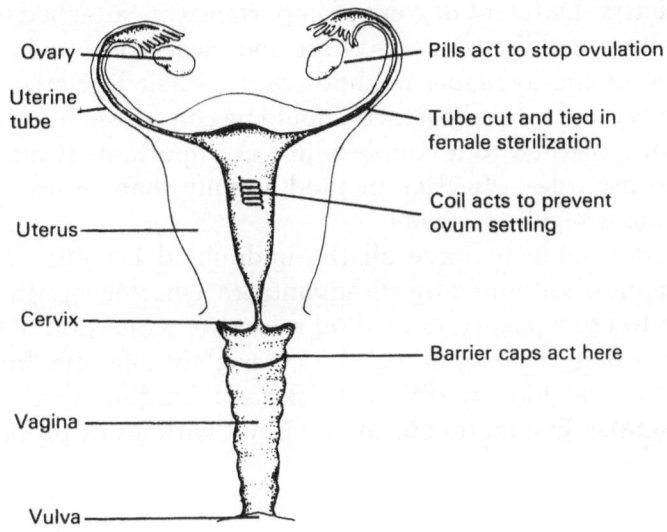

Figure 2.3   Female genital tract seen from the front (showing sites of action of different contraceptives).

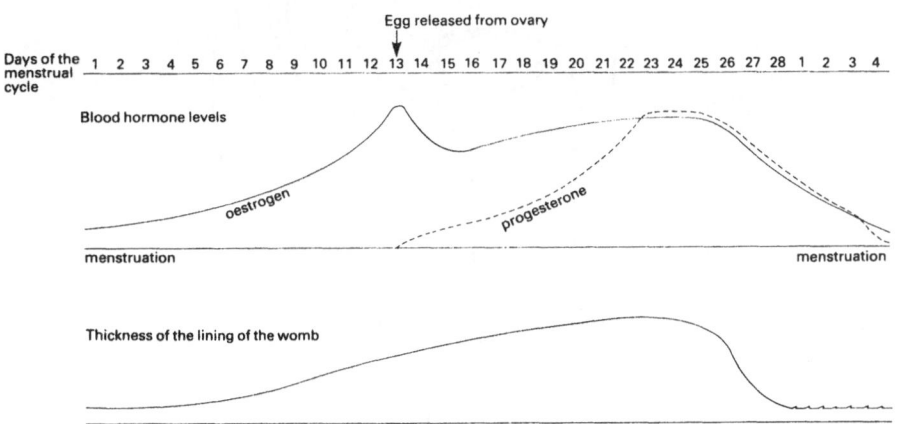

Figure 2.4   The process of menstruation.

Methods of contraception

When deciding on which method of contraception to use the main factors to take into account are those of convenience, safety, and effectiveness. Different degrees of importance are attached to each of these factors at different times of life and most women will use more than one of the available methods during their lifetimes. Before a decision is reached medical facts should be considered but the acceptability of a method to a couple is just as important. It may well be better to use a less-effective method happily than to use a method which causes niggling doubts.

It is impossible to have all the undoubted benefits of modern contraception without any disadvantages whatsoever. In deciding whether to use a particular method it is never a question of choosing between a dangerous option and a completely safe one, but more a question of weighing up different risks and deciding which ones you prefer to take. Even total abstinence is not without its problems.

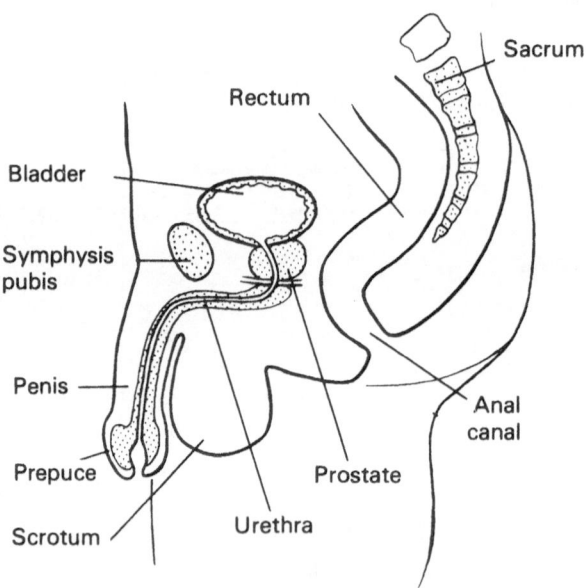

Figure 2.5 Male genital tract seen from the side (see also Figure 2.11, p. 35)

Table 2.3 Effectiveness and times of usage of contraceptive methods

Method	Effectiveness	When best used
Abstinence	100% while adhered to	When wish to make the heart grow fonder.
Sterilization	Virtually 100%	Once sure family is complete.
Pill	Virtually 100%	Below the age of 35 Before and during marriage when wish to be certain no pregnancy will occur If woman suffers from any condition which the pill will benefit or relieve.
Coil	Highly effective	Alternative to the pill for those women who have had at least one child Alternative to sterilization for those coming off the pill For the forgetful.
Progesterone-only pill	Highly effective	Those over 35 who do not wish to be sterilized While breast feeding.
Diaphragm and chemicals	Highly effective	Anyone who cannot or does not wish to take the pill and does not mind slight risk of pregnancy.
Sheath	Highly effective	Where a couple wishes the man to take responsibility for contraception While breast feeding As for the diaphragm.
Withdrawal	Ineffective	Best avoided.
Rhythm	Ineffective	Best avoided.
Douching	Ineffective	May actually increase pregnancy rate.
Breast feeding	Effective	When giving at least six feeds on demand daily. Once less than this or weaning, ovulation will occur within 14—30 days.
None	Ineffective — 80% of women will conceive within one year.	

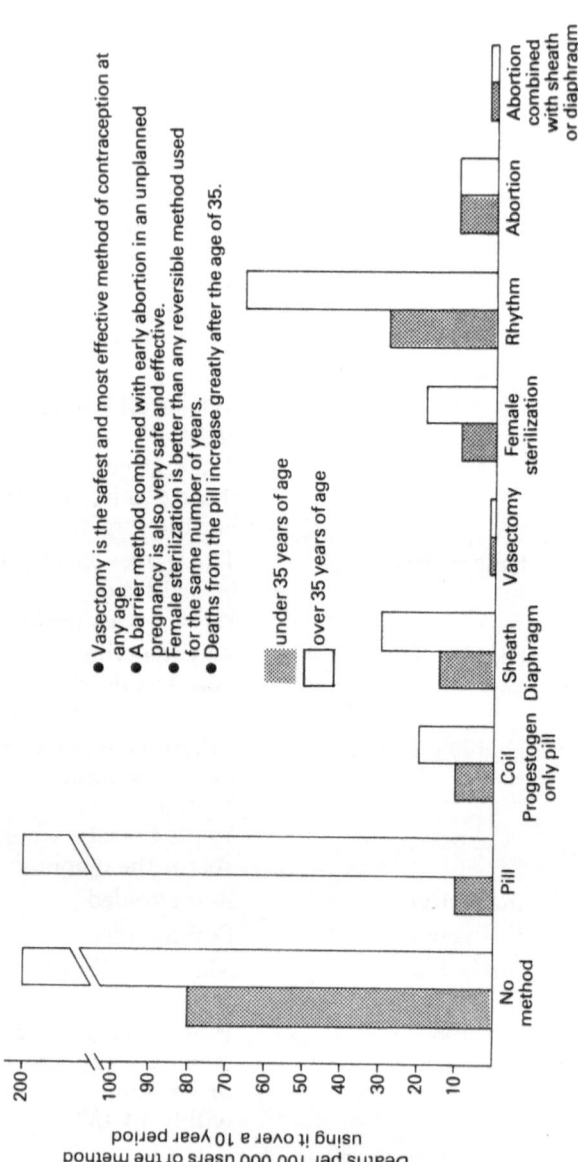

Figure 2.6 Comparison of risks of death from various methods of contraception. (These crude comparisons are subject to many limitations and are meant only as a rough guide.)

When comparing the safety (as measured by risk of death; see Figure 2.6) of contraceptive methods there are two major factors to consider:

the number of deaths caused by the method itself;
the number of deaths that would occur from the unwanted pregnancies that result from failures of the method.

Highly efficient contraceptive methods (the pill, sterilization, and abortion) give rise to very few unwanted pregnancies and so most of their associated deaths are caused by the method itself. Inefficient contraceptive methods, on the other hand, do not directly cause any deaths but cause far more unwanted pregnancies which, apart from the misery and family upset they may cause, lead to proportionately more deaths from pregnancy complications.

Table 2.4 Number of unwanted pregnancies that would occur in a woman using the same method for all her reproductive life (34 years)

Method	No.
Sterilization	None
The pill	None
The coil	Possibly 1
Progesterone-only pill	Possibly 1
The diaphragm	1
The sheath	1–2
Withdrawal	4–5
Rhythm	5
None	13

As can be seen from Table 2.4 and Figure 2.6 the use of no contraception at all is more risky than the use of any of the methods; the less effective a method is (except the pill in those aged over 35) then the more danger there is from it.

Apart from deaths, illness and disease from contraception have to be considered. Again, the amount of illness caused by contraceptive methods is negligible compared with the amount that would be caused by the pregnancies the methods prevent. So, while the most effective methods may cause some illness directly, the ineffective methods may cause more from the unplanned pregnancies that occur as the results of their failure. Complications of individual methods are discussed in detail in the appropriate parts of this chapter.

The pill

Millions of women in Britain and the USA take the pill and there is no doubt that it is a simple, acceptable, and highly effective method of birth control. Despite the fact that it has been more thoroughly studied and more widely used than almost any other medicine the media seem to take a savage delight in giving disproportionate publicity to its real or imagined dangers. It does have side effects and possible complications and it is not suitable for everyone; but the low-dose oestrogen pills now in use are very safe, especially when compared with the risks of pregnancy.

The contraceptive pill contains synthetically produced hormones. Most contain oestrogen and progesterone; some contain only progesterone. Most pills now have 50 micrograms (μg) or less of oestrogen and those with 30 μg or less are known as low-dose pills. They should not be confused with the 'minipill', which has no oestrogen at all. The oestrogen has the main birth-control effect and causes most of the side effects and complications, while the progesterone controls the amount of bleeding in the cycle.

A new triphasic pill just marketed has even lower total hormone doses and may well prove to be safer still, with no loss of effectiveness.

Some questions

Is it safe for me to take the pill? (see Figure 2.7)
For most women the answer to this question will be *yes*, but there are several disorders which can be made worse by the pill and where the pill is therefore contraindicated.

A woman should not take the pill if she has or has had any of the following:

Thrombophlebitis or thrombosis or embolism.
Heart disease or a stroke.
Liver disease, especially hepatitis or jaundice in pregnancy.

Cancer of the uterus, breast, or ovary.
High blood pressure.
High blood fat concentrations.
Less than four periods a year (if you want future pregnancies, as
the pill could stop periods coming altogether).

All these conditions may either be caused or aggravated by the
hormones, especially the oestrogen, in the pill. Anyone who has or has
had any serious illness or who takes any drugs or medicines regularly
should mention this to their physician before starting to take the pill.

These potentially serious conditions are rare. More common
contraindications to taking the pill may be obesity, and heavy
cigarette smoking in women aged over 35.

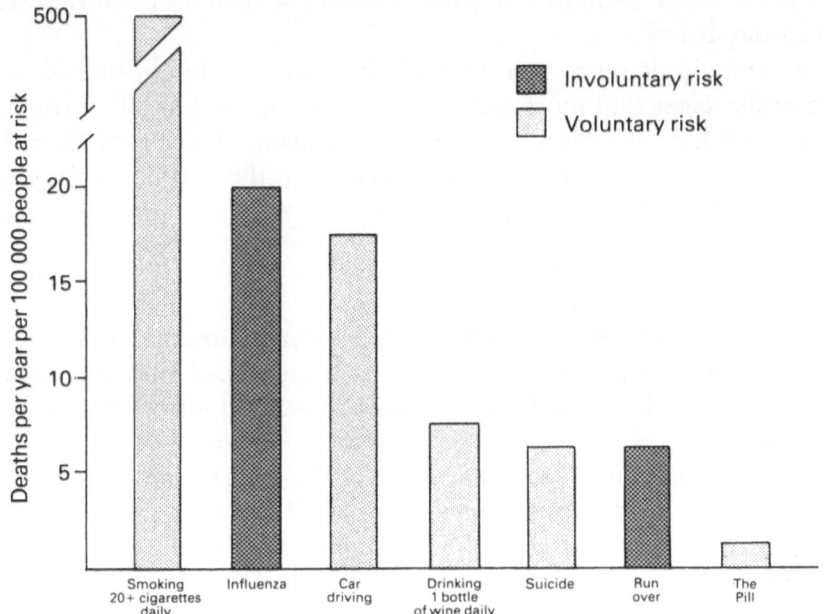

Based on the total sales of the two products, one
cigarette is three times as dangerous to life as
one Pill tablet.

Figure 2.7 The risk of taking the pill put into perspective.

What examination should be carried out before starting the pill?
The physician should know about or will ask about illnesses that have

occurred in the past (but do not assume he or she does). He or she will also ask about the menstrual cycle and when the last period started.

He or she should check blood pressure and note weight and may well want to do an internal (vaginal) pelvic examination and check the breasts for lumps.

Some physicians might take the opportunity to do a smear test, though cancer of the cervix is not connected with the pill.

When do I start taking the pill?

Start on the evening of the first day of the period and take one pill at the same time each day for 21 days, until the packet is finished. Stop taking the pill for 7 days. During this time vaginal blood loss will occur. However light this may be, the next packet must be started after the 7-day break.

As some pills differ, the maker's instructions should be followed carefully. Note that most recommend starting the first pill of the first course on the fifth day of the period and using other precautions for the next 2 weeks; we recommend starting on the first day and not to worry about taking other precautions.

What if I forget to take one?

Take it as soon as remembered unless the gap is more than 12 hours, in which case do not take the one that has been missed but take the next one at the usual time and use additional precautions until the next pill cycle starts.

If you have vomiting or diarrhoea lasting more than a few hours, then again use additional precautions until the next pill cycle. The reason for this is that the pill's hormones may well not have been absorbed adequately from the bowel into the bloodstream and so may not be giving effective contraceptive control.

What are the likely side effects of the pill?

Mild discomforts such as breast tenderness, nausea, bloating, or dizziness may occur in the first month or two but generally disappear after that. Periods will be lighter and in some cases may be missed altogether, although there may be bleeding in the middle of the month.

This is known as 'breakthrough bleeding' and occurs when there is not enough progesterone to keep the lining of the womb intact until the time of the genuine period.

Depression, weight gain (especially before periods), headaches, loss of sex drive, vaginal thrush, discharge from the nipple, and failure of vaginal lubrication may also occur, mainly as a result of the higher oestrogen concentrations in the blood.

What should I do if I experience side effects?
Usually, you should continue taking the pill regardless of any development but if worried about any symptoms then consult your physician. There are a few indications for stopping the pill at once; the decision should be taken by the physician, and the reasons are shown in Table 2.5.

Table 2.5   Possible reasons for stopping the pill

Symptoms	Reason
First ever migraine attack; persistent, severe headache; acute visual disturbance.	May be signs of a developing stroke.
Persistent and unexplained pain in the chest or in a limb.	May be a sign of a developing heart attack or deep-vein thrombosis in the limb.
Development of jaundice.	May be liver inflammation caused or aggravated by the pill.
Known or suspected pregnancy.	Should avoid all drugs in pregnancy; if abortion wanted then the earlier done the better.
Development of phlebitis.	This is caused by the pill and may lead to thrombosis in the limb, or dissemination of clots to other organs.

Will the pill make my periods regular?
Yes. In many cases it will also make them less painful and lighter. It may help premenstrual tension, benign breast disease, endometriosis, acne, and anaemia by changing the hormone balance in the body.

Does the pill cause cancer?
No. The pill probably reduces the risk of developing cancer of the ovary and uterus.

What are the risks of serious complications occurring?
Deep-vein thrombosis is clotting of blood in the veins (usually of the legs) and occurs four times more often in a pill user than in a non-user. It is not dangerous if it stays in the limb but if a large clot breaks off and stops in the lungs (embolism) then the outcome may be fatal.

Phlebitis is redness, pain, and tenderness round the surface veins of the legs and occurs 2—3 times more often than in a non-user. It is also more likely in women with bad varicose veins. It can be very sore but poses no danger to life.

Raised blood pressure is noted in up to 5% of users after 5 years on the pill. It may be caused by oestrogen affecting the walls of blood vessels and is similar to the blood pressure rise that can occur in pregnancy. In nearly all cases the blood pressure goes back to normal when the pill is stopped.

Heart attacks/strokes show an increased incidence in pill takers, particularly in those over the age of 35 and even more particularly in those that also smoke. The risk of a heart attack from the pill alone is one half that of a woman not taking the pill who smokes. A WOMAN WHO SMOKES AND TAKES THE PILL HAS HER CHANCES OF HAVING A HEART ATTACK INCREASED BY 20 TIMES. If you cannot stop smoking then certainly once you are over the age of 35 you should stop taking the pill.

Will the pill reduce my chances of getting pregnant in the future?
No. Except temporarily (for a few months) in about 2% of women who have had no children.

What regular checks should my physician do when I am on the pill?
The only medical examination required specifically for the care of a woman on the pill is a blood pressure check once or twice a year. The physician will want to make sure you are not putting on weight and may well do an internal examination and a smear test every 3—5 years.

How often should I have a cervical smear test carried out?
Smear tests are designed to examine the cells of the neck of the womb to see if any are abnormal and at risk of developing into cancer cells. Only about 30% of women with these abnormal cells would actually develop cancer and in most of them this process would take about 8—10 years. However, by finding the abnormal cells and removing them the chance of a woman getting cancer of the cervix is reduced.

A first smear test should be done when a woman is in her 20s with a check one year later, then every 5 years until she reaches the age of 35, and three yearly after that.

When should I stop taking the pill?
The risks of serious problems with the pill, though still small, increase once a woman passes the age of 35 and from then on other methods should be considered. Smokers should be prepared to stop taking the pill from the age of 30 onwards.

There is no medical reason to have breaks while taking the pill but it should be stopped one month before going into hospital for any planned operation and obviously when you want to get pregnant. When it is stopped there may be a one-period or two-period gap between the last pill-induced period and the first completely natural one — this is known as post-pill amenorrhoea and is of no consequence.

Should I have a blood test for German measles (rubella) before I ever want to get pregnant?
Yes. German measles or rubella is difficult to diagnose clinically so many women who assume they have had it may not have done, and some who believe they have not had it may have done. About one in five women in the reproductive age group are not rubella immune. If they are infected in early pregnancy (the first 12 weeks especially) then there is a high chance of the baby developing severe congenital abnormalities. Indeed, if rubella occurs in the first 8 weeks of pregnancy then there is only about a one in three chance of an absolutely normal baby being born.

By a simple blood test the physician can tell whether a woman has immunity to rubella or not. If she has not then immunization can be carried out — after making sure she is not pregnant at the time and that she will not get pregnant for the next 12 weeks. Only one injection is needed.

No one pill formulation suits all women because of the interplay between the woman's natural hormones and the type and amount of hormones in the pill. While most women will find their first pill suitable some may need to try more than one different brand. When changing brands the first of the new ones should be taken the day after the last of the old ones and, in that way, no additional contraception will be needed.

If for any reason you do not wish to have a period at the time it is due then carry on with another pill packet without taking the 7-day break.

The progesterone-only pill (minipill)

This contains synthetic progesterone only and has far fewer side effects and complications than the combined pill. It is less effective as a contraceptive. It can cause breast tenderness, weight gain, and depression but the main problem with its use is irregularity of the periods, especially in the first few months. There are no serious side effects but there is an increased risk of pregnancy.

It should be started on the first day of a period and taken every day from then on — without any breaks. Extra precautions need to be taken for the first 14 days; for 14 days if the taking of a tablet is forgotten; and for 14 days if you have vomiting or diarrhoea.

The coil (intrauterine device; IUD)

About 8% of women using contraception in Britain and the USA are fitted with coils and they accept the slight risk of pregnancy and possible side effects in return for the convenience the method offers.

All the side effects are more likely to occur in younger, childless women and — as an infection from the coil can give rise to infertility — coils are best used in women who have had children.

What side effects may occur?
About one in ten coils will be expelled from the womb, especially in the first few months.

About one in ten coils may need to be removed because of heavy or painful periods. Anaemia may be caused or aggravated.

Pelvic infection may occur in about one in fifty women and may cause subsequent infertility.

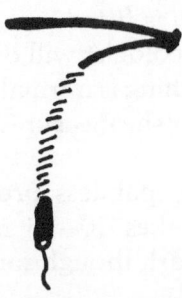

Figure 2.8   The Copper-7 IUD. This is a small, copper-containing coil which lasts two years then needs changing; there are fewer side effects than with plastic coils but it is more likely to fall out.

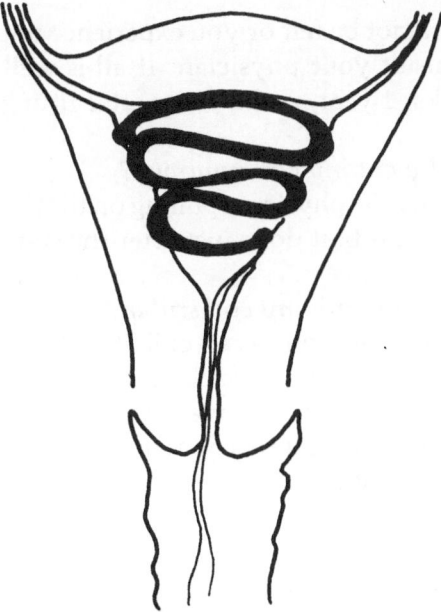

Figure 2.9   The Lippes loop *in situ*. This is a larger, plastic coil which may need to be changed after 8—10 years; there are more side effects than with copper coils.

Will my physician fit the coil?
Apart from gynaecologists, many family physicians fit coils but if they do not, yet think the coil would suit you, then they can soon arrange for another to do it.

What happens when the coil is fitted?
First the physician or gynaecologist will do an internal and speculum examination to check everything is normal. Then he or she will leave a speculum in place while he or she measures the inside of the womb and then fits the coil.

This should be a simple, painless procedure. No anaesthetic is necessary and the fitting takes 10—15 minutes. Most women are surprised at how little they feel, though some may experience cramps.

What check-ups should be done after the coil is fitted?
When the coil is in the womb, threads (like cotton) hang down into the vagina and can be felt there. They can be checked there regularly by self-examination.

If the threads cannot be felt or you experience undue pain or heavy bleeding then consult your physician. If all is well have the coil re-checked in 6 weeks, 1 year, and 2 years after fitting.

What happens if I want my coil removed?
This is easily done by the physician pulling on the threads. It takes only a minute or two and is best done just after the start of a period.

What if I get pregnant with my coil still in?
If a period is missed while you have a coil fitted then check by having a pregnancy test and seeing the physician. If you wish the pregnancy to continue then the coil may be removed (at hospital). There is a greater chance of a miscarriage but, if this does not happen, there are no extra risks to the unborn child.

The male sheath

Originally designed to prevent its user from catching venereal disease (VD) rather than as a contraceptive, the sheath is effective provided it is used properly every time intercourse takes place.

It must be put on when the penis is erect and before any penetration takes place (sperms can come out of the penis before ejaculation occurs). Any air in the top of the sheath must be expelled as the sheath is unrolled over the penis (this helps prevent the sheath bursting during ejaculation). After ejaculation the sheath should be held close to the penis so that it remains in place until the penis has been withdrawn. Withdrawal should take place while the penis is still erect so that there is no risk of the sheath slipping off and allowing semen into the vagina. Use of chemical foam or pessaries with the sheath increases its effectiveness.

The diaphragm (see Figure 2.10)

Like the sheath the diaphragm (cap) has no side effects and is a very underrated method. It requires conscientiousness and organization as the onus is on the user to take correct action before intercourse. If put in every night (whether needed or not) it takes about as much time as brushing one's teeth and allows spontaneous intercourse to take place.

There is evidence that the incidence of cancer of the cervix is reduced by using the diaphragm (and presumably the sheath).

It has to be initially fitted by a physician or gynaecologist, though a new one-sized one that requires no medical supervision is being tested.

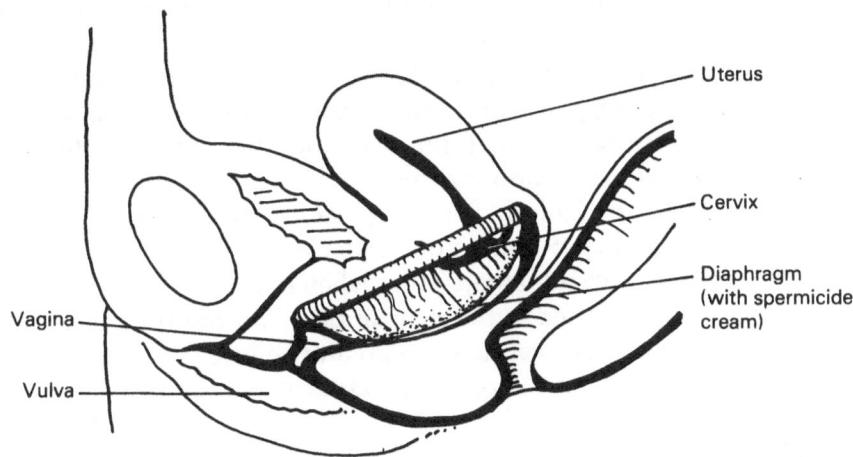

Figure 2.10 A diaphragm, used with spermicide inside it.

Withdrawal

Known also as *coitus interruptus*, this method relies on the man withdrawing the erect penis before orgasm and ejaculation take place. As sperms can pass out of the penis before ejaculation takes place and as it is often very difficult to stop in time, this method is unreliable. It requires a degree of self-control which is unlikely to be acquired without considerable experience and risk of pregnancy. It also leads to frustration, especially on the part of the woman, and can therefore give rise to marital problems.

Rhythm

This method of contraception depends on avoiding sexual intercourse around the time of ovulation, when conception is most likely to occur. It is termed 'natural' by its protagonists but it is more natural than any other form of contraception only in so far as it does least to thwart nature's aim of maximum reproduction.

Ovulation can occur at any time in the cycle and possibly more than once in some cycles as a direct response to the stimulation of intercourse. There is no foolproof way of discovering when ovulation is about to occur, although by taking a daily temperature and feeling vaginal secretions it usually can be determined when it actually occurs. Intercourse has to be avoided until ovulation occurs and for 3 days after. Making all allowances for possible times of ovulation will usually give a 'safe' period of 11 days or so in any month. Intercourse therefore can take place only on those days, despite the woman's increased sex drive at other times in the cycle and whatever the couple's natural inclination may be.

Even with a tremendous amount of motivation, self-control, and mathematical ability it is still not a reliable method of contraception and has the added disadvantages that when unplanned pregnancies do occur they have started with fertilization of an old (possibly dying) egg. This means there is probably a greater chance of miscarriage and possibly an increase in the risk of an abnormal baby being born.

Sterilization

When a woman has reached her early 30s most families have been completed and most women have a further 15—20 years of fertility ahead of them during which they will need contraception. Any reversible method used in older women for this length of time is going to cause considerable problems and be far more dangerous than steril-ization. The pill — which is the only method with a similar degree of effectiveness — is associated, at this age, with a great increase in deaths (from the method itself) while the level of unplanned pregnancies with other methods is far less acceptable than it might have been when the woman was younger. An unwanted pregnancy in a 25-year-old with one child is not the same kind of disaster that an unwanted pregnancy would be in a 42-year-old whose youngest child is 17.

Vasectomy

This simple operation to divide the vas deferens (hence 'vasectomy' — to cut the vas) is generally done under local anaesthetic and takes about 15—20 minutes. Until there are two negative sperm tests (performed at 12 and 16 weeks after the operation) alternative contraception has to be used. After that the operation should be considered successful and irreversible.

Bruising, swelling, and infection are possible complications from the operation, but there is no evidence in man of any long-term complications whatsoever. It is the safest of all the contraceptive methods, causing little illness and virtually no deaths.

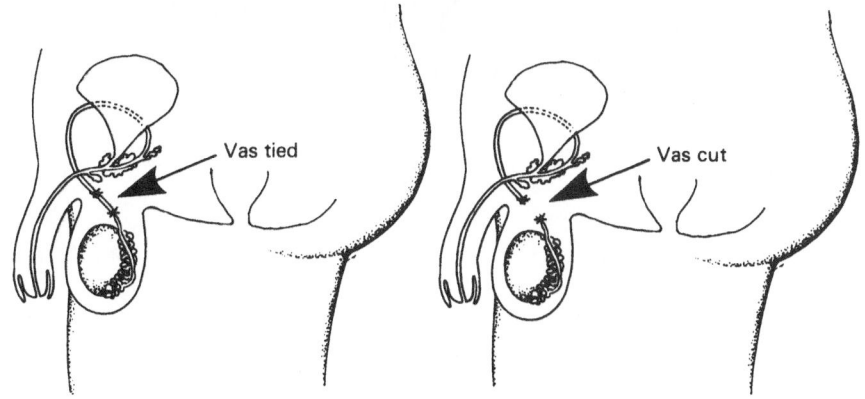

Figure 2.11   How a vasectomy is performed.

After the operation sexual desire, sexual response, erection, orgasm, and ejaculation all occur completely normally. The only difference is that there are no sperms in the ejaculated fluid. While no sexual problems will result from the operation no one should undergo vasectomy if they already have sexual problems or if they are not completely happy about it.

Female sterilization

This is done either by opening the abdomen and dividing the Fallopian tubes (mini-laparotomy) or with an instrument called a laparoscope, which is passed into the abdomen through a cut ½−1 inch long below the navel (umbilicus) and allows the gynaecologist to see and cut the Fallopian tubes by remote control.

Laparoscopic sterilization is immediate, permanent, and should be regarded as irreversible. It requires a general anaesthetic and there are approximately 8 deaths per 100 000 operations. Recognized long-term complications include heavy periods, cramping pains and, more rarely, depression and bowel obstruction from adhesions.

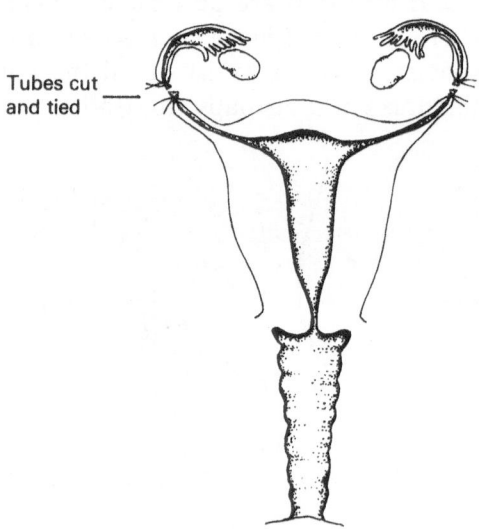

Tubes cut
and tied

Figure 2.12   Female sterilization: cutting and tying uterine tubes.

Before sterilization the couple must be absolutely certain that they want no more children regardless of what might happen to the marriage, the partner, or any existing children.

Abortion

120 000 pregnancies are terminated in Britain each year and 1 400 000 in the USA. Abortion is not a recommended method of birth control but as nearly all methods have some risk of failure abortion is a necessary back-up facility.

The earlier in pregnancy it is carried out the better, as it is then a more minor and safer procedure. After the twelfth week of pregnancy it becomes much more difficult.

In many areas abortion is safest, quickest, and most conveniently carried out in a private clinic or by an abortion charity. However, only your physician can advise on local resources. If he is against abortion or you do not wish him to know, then seek out other local legitimate facilities and approach them directly.

Modern methods of abortion do not weaken the neck of the womb and do not make it more likely that there will be miscarriage in the future, provided that the operation is done before the twelfth week of pregnancy.

Severe psychological disturbance is more common in women who have babies at full term than in those who have abortions. About one in ten women will have severe regrets over abortion compared with about four in ten of those who are refused abortion and later regret having continued the pregnancy.

Normal sex

The pattern of sexual activity within a partnership such as marriage is infinitely varied. No absolute standard of normality can be laid down. 'Normal' is what pleases both partners most and it is different for each couple. Within every relationship, the pattern changes as time passes, ideally giving greater mutual pleasure and satisfaction with increasing love, trust, and maturity.

No relationship runs smoothly throughout its course and it is normal for problems to arise within a sexual relationship. Some of the commonest problems arise from *inexperience and ignorance* of sexual physiology and technique.

It is obvious to everyone that for intercourse to take place the man must have an erect penis. It is less obvious and not universally recognized that a similar process occurs in the woman, making the tissues of the vulva and vagina swollen and tense and lubricated with mucus. This has the effect of protecting the genitalia and cushioning them from trauma during intercourse. It is possible for intercourse to take place without this sexual arousal in the woman but it is not so pleasurable for either partner and may lead to soreness and inflammation of the vagina (vaginitis) or bruising of the urethra (the passage leading from the bladder) and cystitis. If penetration takes place before the woman is fully aroused, she may well reach full arousal later but will be lagging behind her partner and is unlikely to achieve orgasm before he has finished. She may then be left feeling very frustrated.

Many women take longer than their partners to reach the advanced state of arousal necessary for satisfactory intercourse. This need not be a problem as long as it is recognized and understood. It may be overcome by extended foreplay during which the couple explore ways of pleasurably arousing the woman while the man holds back and avoids becoming over-stimulated. Spending the earlier part of the evening together, watching an erotic film, dancing and petting may all have a similar result. Fatigue, anxiety, anger, and resentment all inhibit sexual arousal in women.

Sexual myths

Much sexual anxiety arises from the mass of myths and traditions which pervade society. These concern the size of the genitalia, normal positions and frequency of intercourse, the effects of masturbation, and many others. To mention a few:

The size of the penis is unimportant. The smaller the penis before erection, the greater the degree of enlargement when erect. The intensity of pleasure derived from intercourse by the woman is not related to the size of the penis.

The apparent size of the vagina is unimportant. The walls are folded and very elastic and expand to contain any size of erect penis. It is, after all, designed for the passage of a baby's head!

Masturbation never does any harm.

The best position for intercourse is whatever the couple enjoy most. Many couples change position during intercourse and use different positions on different occasions.

The frequency of intercourse depends entirely on individual feelings. It will vary from one couple to another and in the same couple at different times. What is normal for a newly married couple with no children will be unthinkable when the same couple has a new baby or reaches middle age. Comparing notes with friends is disastrous. Everyone is different. There is no standard norm.

Ranges and variations

It is natural for sex drive (libido) to be reduced in a woman who has just had a child and this may last for a year or more. It is nature's contraceptive. It is also natural for libido to lessen with increasing age, although it may increase when the children leave home, when the couple are on holiday, or when an anxiety is relieved — for instance, after sterilization.

It is inevitable that partners will sometimes have different appetites for intercourse. As in all other aspects of the relationship, what they do will be a compromise. A woman who has recently had a baby may find herself sometimes having intercourse because she loves her husband and wants to please him rather than because she herself is keen to. Similarly he will sometimes be prepared to suppress his own desires rather than persuade her to comply when she really does not feel like it.

The most satisfying sexual experiences occur within a stable, loving relationship with good communication between the partners. This applies to both partners but it is particularly difficult for a woman to desire intercourse and achieve sexual arousal and orgasm if the relationship is going through a bad patch in other areas. It may sometimes appear that marital difficulties are arising from a woman's lack of enthusiasm for sex, when in fact it is the other way round. If the marriage is going well, sex should come right.

It may be difficult for couples to sort out problems for themselves and the usefulness and importance of marriage counselling is now well recognized. The marriage guidance council, family planning clinics, and some churches provide valuable services.

3
Pregnancy

Pregnancy is the physiological process whereby the fertilized ovum develops within the mother until the fetus is ready to live an independent existence as a baby.

The aims of antenatal care, supervision of labour, and postnatal care are:

1. To ensure the health and safety of the mother.
2. To facilitate the live birth of a full-term, normal baby, without congenital or developmental abnormality.
3. To help both the mother and the father achieve the knowledge and capacity to provide for the physical, emotional, and social needs of the baby.

It may be argued that since pregnancy and labour are normal physiological processes no help or supervision is required. After all, nature has done the job perfectly well for thousands of years, has she not? Whilst it may well be true that, as far as the whole species, *Homo sapiens*, is concerned, the wastage of fetal and maternal life may be biologically acceptable, it is clearly unacceptable in human terms that preventable causes of death and malformation of infants, and risks to the life or health of the mother should be tolerated.

Maternal mortality has shown a dramatic decline in all developed countries over the past fifty years (Figure 3.1). The most striking fall initially was a dramatic reduction in deaths due to infections. This

41

problem was largely overcome by introducing sterile techniques, anti-biotics, and sulphonamide drugs. Another important development in medical care available to pregnant women was the increasing availability of blood transfusion services from the time of the second world war. Also at this time, the concept of antenatal clinics where abnormalities of pregnancy could be detected and treated was gaining acceptance. And the general level of maternal health and nutrition improved considerably, together with improvements in housing and other social conditions.

The very small number of maternal deaths which occur today in developed countries are intensively investigated to discover whether any opportunities for prevention had been missed during pregnancy or labour. In some 40% of cases avoidable factors are demonstrated and action taken to correct them.

Perinatal mortality refers to the number of babies who are stillborn after the 28th week of pregnancy or who die in the first week of life. This figure has also dropped dramatically over the past fifty years from over 100 in every 1000 births in 1925 in the developed nations to a rate of below 20 per 1000 births today. There is evidence from many

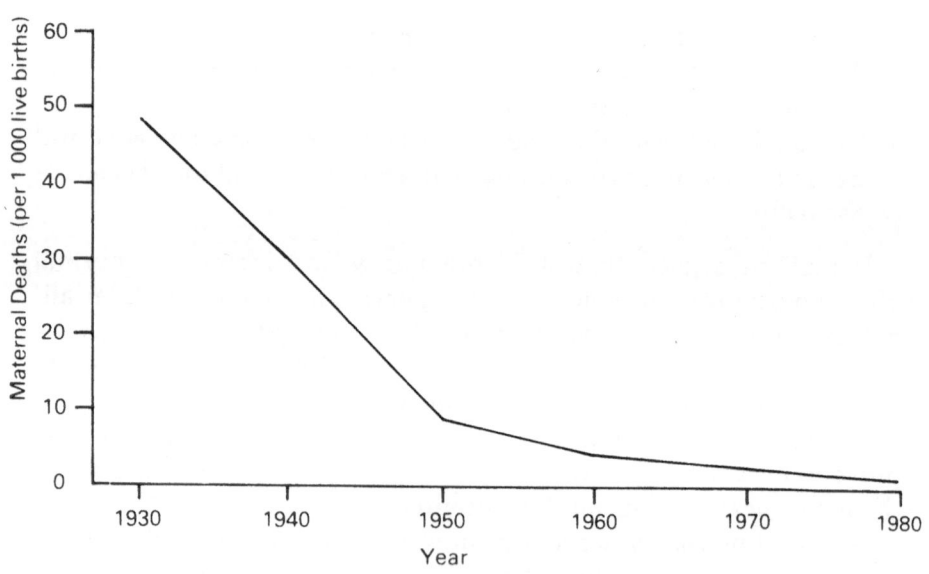

Figure 3.1   Maternal mortality in UK, 1930–1980.

countries that more infants could be saved by the better application of existing knowledge and the better organization of existing medical services.

However, it has become increasingly clear that both maternal and perinatal mortality are most closely linked with the social circumstances of the mother. Married women between the ages of 20 and 30 years, from the higher social classes, not smoking, and bearing not more than four children have the least likelihood of a complicated pregnancy and labour, whilst less fortunate women and their children face higher risks.

Thus, society must endeavour to provide the nutritional, housing, employment, educational, and medical services which favour good health, whilst the individual patient must accept some degree of monitoring of, and at times intervention in, the normal physiological process of pregnancy and labour. However, it is well to bear in mind that technical improvements in care should not be introduced wholesale without considering the effects on the emotional and human aspects of childbearing. A compromise has to be found between providing, as unobtrusively as possible, good technical care, whilst at the same time providing a suitable social and emotional environment for the family and the new baby.

Who does what?

During the course of pregnancy a woman is likely to come into contact with several types of professional worker. It can sometimes be confusing and difficult to sort out who is who and who does what.

In the UK these people include midwives, health visitors, general practitioners, and obstetricians and some families also will need the help of a social worker.

The *midwife* is a nurse with special training in all aspects of pregnancy and labour. In the UK he or she is usually the person primarily responsible for supervision of pregnancy and management of labour in the normal, uncomplicated case.

The *health visitor* (public health nurse) is specially trained in the social and emotional aspects of pregnancy and child care, with a focus on the maintenance of health and the prevention of illness.

The *general practitioner* (family physician) is a generalist with a wide range of expertise, including obstetric care. General practitioners vary in the amount of training they have undertaken in obstetrics and in the degree of interest, enthusiasm, and continuing practical experience which they have for this field of work. Accordingly, a few general practitioners will confine their care to diagnosing pregnancy and managing any intercurrent illness, whilst others will play a larger part in routine antenatal and postnatal care. The work of general practitioners in the management of labour and delivery is decreasing in the UK, but nevertheless many uncomplicated deliveries in hospital and all home deliveries still remain the responsibility of the family physician and the midwife.

The *specialist obstetrician* is based in a hospital or clinic, and in most developed countries almost all babies are born in hospitals or clinics. In Britain the role of the specialist obstetrician and his or her team is to provide direct care and supervision for patients with actual or potential medical and obstetric problems, and to provide support and advice in any case where the physician or midwife requests help.

High-quality care depends on a close relationship between the professionals concerned, so that the patient should receive that level of care which is required at a given moment. It is expensive, wasteful and often a social inconvenience to the patient if highly specialized care is provided for patients who have no need of it. Nevertheless, this is the established pattern in private obstetric practice all over the world. The concept of 'shared care', in which the various professionals co-operate appropriately in the care of each patient, has been developed very considerably in the UK over the past 15 years.

The course of pregnancy

Traditionally, pregnancy is divided into three trimesters, or periods of three months. During the first trimester large hormonal changes occur as the woman's body adjusts itself to the new experience of pregnancy. The second trimester is a more settled phase of growth and development whilst, in the third trimester, the mother's body is prepared for delivery and subsequent lactation.

The first trimester (0—13 weeks)
Diagnosis of pregnancy
The features of early pregnancy, of which most women are aware, are

listed in Table 3.1. The earliest moment at which it is worthwhile consulting a physician is about six weeks after the first day of the last menstrual period. This is the time at which the immunological hormone pregnancy test on urine (a HCG test) becomes reliably positive if the patient is pregnant. However, in most cases it is probably better to wait until two menstrual periods have been missed and 8—9 weeks have elapsed since the last period because, at this stage, the physician can usually check by examination alone that the uterus is softened and definitely enlarged.

Table 3.1   Early features of pregnancy

Period missed or abnormally light.
Feeling of sickness, especially in the morning (can last up to 16 weeks).
Breast tingling, soreness, swelling (from 6 weeks).
Secretion from the nipple and pigmentation of the areola (from 12 weeks).
Frequent passing of urine (8—14 weeks).
Constipation may become troublesome.
Increased clear vaginal discharge.
Blue or purple discoloration of the vaginal walls.

Drugs in early pregnancy
Since the thalidomide tragedy most women and their physicians have become acutely aware of the dangers of taking drugs in early pregnancy. Even drugs which have been extensively used for many years to combat nausea and sickness have come under suspicion of damaging the embryo and giving rise to a congenitally malformed baby.

In view of the controversy which surrounds the subject the only advice must be never to take any drug in early pregnancy unless it is absolutely essential.

Counselling before pregnancy
If a patient is already taking a drug for a long-standing condition such as diabetes or epilepsy then it is wise for her to consult a physician as early as possible, preferably before embarking on a pregnancy. Indeed, any patient who suffers from a serious medical or gynaecological condition would be well advised to do likewise.

German measles (rubella)

Ideally, no woman should embark upon a pregnancy without having first had a blood test to confirm that she is immune to the disease. If she has no antibodies to protect her then immunization with rubella vaccine will provide the necessary security provided that she avoids pregnancy for three months afterwards.

If a woman is not sure whether she is immune to rubella and she believes that she may have been in contact with the disease in early pregnancy, then she should contact her physician as soon as possible so that a blood test may be performed. If she is not immune then a further blood test three weeks later will determine whether or not she has contracted the disease. It is not possible to rely on the woman developing the typical signs of the disease, a rash and swollen glands, since infection can occur without the patient becoming ill, and since other viruses can produce an identical illness with no risk to the baby.

If proven rubella infection occurs in the first trimester, and especially before eight weeks of pregnancy, then the chances of the infant surviving completely undamaged are less than one in three. The baby may have a damaged brain causing mental retardation, deafness or blindness, congenital defects of the heart, or a multitude of less serious abnormalities. In these unfortunate cases the option of terminating the pregnancy must be seriously considered.

Bleeding in early pregnancy

Bleeding in early pregnancy is a common problem. It may, of course, merely represent a late or otherwise abnormal period if the patient has not been proved to be pregnant, or if it occurs at the time of an expected period it may represent the normal pattern for some women who continue to have some monthly bleeding for the first two or three months of pregnancy. However, if the patient is pregnant, any bleeding in early pregnancy must be regarded as abnormal unless proved otherwise, since it usually represents a *threatened miscarriage*. Natural miscarriages are common. At least one in every six pregnancies ends in a miscarriage, and probably many more which occur so early that the patient may not be aware that she was pregnant.

The most likely cause is some abnormality of the embryo which is incompatible with life and must be regarded as nature's way of preventing a biological disaster. However, in a few women recurrent miscarriages occur and may be due to structural or hormonal problems. There is no evidence that a normal fetus can be dislodged by lifting, falling, sexual intercourse, riding a bicycle, or swimming the English Channel! Neither is there any good evidence that complete bed rest or injections of hormones in early pregnancy prevent recurrent miscarriages; indeed, the hormones may possibly be harmful.

Whilst many pregnancies continue normally to term without ill effects after a threatened miscarriage, special supervision is indicated since the placental function may be inadequate later in pregnancy. Usually, *threatened miscarriage* is painless. If severe, period-like cramp pain develops and bleeding increases the miscarriage becomes *inevitable* and will either occur spontaneously with the loss of the products of conception or remain *incomplete* in which case hospital admission for surgical evacuation of the uterus is indicated.

Very rarely, lower abdominal pain is the predominant symptom and precedes vaginal bleeding. This may indicate an *ectopic pregnancy*; that is, a pregnancy developing outside the uterus in one of the Fallopian tubes. This is a serious condition which requires prompt hospital admission for confirmation of the diagnosis and surgical treatment, because if untreated severe internal bleeding may occur from erosion of blood vessels by the growing ovum.

Antenatal care — 'The booking attendance'
After pregnancy has been confirmed the patient will be seen again to make all the necessary arrangements for the pregnancy. This *booking attendance* may take place at the physician's office or at the hospital antenatal clinic. Wherever the consultation the routine will be similar. The doctor or nurse will ask the patient about her previous medical, gynaecological, and obstetric history, searching for clues which may point to potential problems. He or she will endeavour to uncover any hidden anxieties regarding pregnancy and labour and provide appropriate counselling or referral for further help if required. Table 3.2 indicates general advice for pregnancy.

A general examination to detect medical problems is normally undertaken, as is a pelvic examination to determine the size and position of the uterus and to detect any problems such as fibroids or an ovarian cyst which may cause troubles later in pregnancy. The patient is weighed, the blood pressure measured, and a urine specimen tested.

Finally, a specimen of blood is taken from an arm vein. Usually the results of all these investigations are recorded on a co-operation card, which is kept by the patient throughout her pregnancy. The meaning and significance of the terms used and the notes recorded are shown in Table 3.3.

Table 3.2   General advice for pregnancy

Dress	Wear comfortable, loose-fitting clothes. Beware of high heels. Choose a well-fitting bra to give maximum breast support.
Diet	Increase intake of fluid and roughage (fresh fruit, vegetables, brown bread, bran cereals, etc.) well above normal to prevent constipation. Eat extra meat or fish for first-class protein and at least 1 pint (0.57 l) of milk per day for protein, calcium, and phosphorus.
Alcohol	Not harmful in moderation.
Smoking	Increases risk of premature birth and baby dying.
Nipples	Retracted nipples may be drawn out daily with the fingers to help prepare for breast feeding. Soap and water for cleaning; no other special care needed.
Exercise	Moderate exercise at all stages may be beneficial. Violent exercise best avoided, particularly if there is a history of miscarriage (avoid before 14 weeks especially).
Travel	Try to avoid sitting still in one place for too long at a time; otherwise commonsense should be used.
Work	As long as you feel like it, except possibly in the last month.
Sexual intercourse	Not a hazard to mother or baby either from thrusting or infection. May well need to change position but can take place throughout pregnancy and as soon after delivery as inclination dictates provided there is no history of bleeding in pregnancy, no risk of premature labour, the membranes have not broken, and it does not cause vaginal or abdominal pain.
Drugs	Best avoided at all stages, especially during the first 16 weeks unless mother needs them for medical condition. Paracetamol, kaolin, Senokot syrup, anti-sickness tablets (*from doctor*) and simple cough linctuses (e.g. honey or lemon) are safe.

Table 3.3. Guide to the antenatal co-operation card

LMP	Last menstrual period	Taken from first day of last period and forms base line for all calculations of duration of pregnancy.
EDD or EDC	Estimated date of delivery or confinement	Add 9 calendar months plus 1 week to LMP to get rough idea of when baby is due. Medically, pregnancy is 40 weeks long, i.e. 10 × 4 week-long months.
ABO	Main blood group	You are either O (47% of the population); A (43%); B (8%); or AB (2%).
Rh	Rhesus blood group	Rh positive (85% of the population) or Rh negative (15%). Important only if you are Rh negative and your babies are Rh positive. For this the father must be Rh positive.
Antibodies	Rhesus antibodies	These appear in the blood if a Rh-negative mother has been affected by a Rh-positive baby. If they develop then the baby can be harmed by them. These are checked for routinely throughout a Rh-negative woman's pregnancy. Immunization after delivery or miscarriage prevents this problem.
WR/Kahn	Wasserman test	Routine test to exclude syphilis, which if present will affect baby severely but which if found can be easily treated.
Hb	Haemoglobin concentration	This always drops in pregnancy. If below 12 grams (g)/100 ml of blood then needs rechecking; if below 10 g/100 ml then needs treatment.
Wt	Body weight	Not more than 12.7 kg (28 lb) gain in the entire pregnancy, or 2.27 kg (5 lb) in any month. In the first half of pregnancy Mum gains weight and in the second half

(Continued)

Table 3.3   Continued

		baby does. At 6 lunar months baby weighs 0.45 kg (1 lb); at 7 months 0.91 kg (2 lb); at 8 months 1.6 kg (3½ lb), and at 9 months 3.2 kg (7 lb).
Urinalysis	Urine tests	For protein and sugar. Protein may be a sign of urinary infection or of pre-eclampsia (high blood pressure). Sugar quite commonly found; but if it recurs may be sign of diabetes.
BP	Blood pressure	Checked at every visit. Up to 140/90 mm Hg is normal.
Fundus	Size of womb	At 12—13 weeks just felt above pubic bone; at 20 weeks should have reached umbilicus and at 36 weeks fills the abdomen.
Presentation and position		How the baby is lying. Either vertex (Vx), which is head downwards, or breech (Br), which is bottom downwards. Also either free or engaged (after 36 weeks when head drops down into pelvis — only in first pregnancy).
FMF	Fetal movements felt	About 21—22 weeks for first baby and 17—18 or so thereafter. Shows baby is well and kicking.
FH	Fetal heart	Can be heard with a microphone from 14 weeks onwards but not with stethoscope until much later. More important in labour than in antenatal care.
Oedema		Fluid at ankles/fingers which may be sign of pre-eclampsia.
Rubella antibodies		If present this means there is no risk of contracting the disease.
NAD	Nothing abnormal detected	

With the information obtained at the booking clinic the physician is in a position to discuss the most suitable place for delivery. Most births occur in hospital, but home delivery is attracting more attention. Generally speaking, patients for whom a home delivery is suitable are those aged under 35 with no significant medical history and no previous obstetric complications who are having their second or third babies. There is evidence that this group of patients and their babies are at minimum risk. However, no pregnancy and labour can be considered entirely normal, except in retrospect, and it is for this reason that physicians are becoming increasingly reluctant to take responsibility for home deliveries. Whilst home delivery can be a most rewarding and enjoyable family experience, anyone who has tried to cope with an obstetric emergency in the middle of the night with inadequate light, inadequate equipment, and inadequate support is unlikely to wish to repeat the experience. Arrangements whereby the patient can be admitted to hospital in labour, delivered by the district midwife, and returned home with the baby within 24 hours overcome almost all of the usual objections to hospital delivery. In our view we should recreate within the hospital the easy access for the family and the personal contact with the professionals concerned which patients enjoy so much at home. Combined with the extra margin of safety which the hospital affords this seems to us to be a 'best-buy' solution.

New tests in early pregnancy
A new test which has only recently become available is the test for *alphafetoprotein* in the blood. This is a substance produced in excess by certain fetal deformities. This test is gradually becoming a routine procedure. If the concentration of this substance in the blood is raised then there is a strong possibility of a serious congenital disorder of the nervous system such as anencephaly (brain deformity) or spina bifida being present in the fetus. Confirmation requires the procedure known as *amniocentesis*, which cannot be performed until about 16 weeks. A needle is introduced into the uterus through the abdominal wall to remove some of the amniotic fluid surrounding the fetus. If the level of alphafetoprotein in the amniotic fluid is also significantly raised then the diagnosis is almost certain and termination of pregnancy must be considered. Amniocentesis also may allow the detection of chromosomal abnormalities such as mongolism and possibly other congenital

defects in the future. This procedure must not be undertaken lightly, however, since there is a 1% chance of inducing a miscarriage and, of course, there is no point in the investigation if the mother has strong objections to termination of pregnancy in any circumstances, since no corrective treatment is available for these disorders. The tests are indicators for possible termination of the pregnancy to prevent birth of a deformed baby.

A new method of investigation which appears to be entirely safe is the *ultrasonic scan*. This technique, which is painless and harmless, consists of applying a small transmitter of ultrasonic waves to the mother's abdomen. These ultrasonic waves are reflected from the contents of the abdomen and the uterus and may be received and displayed on a screen. The principle is similar to that of an echo-sounder for detecting submarines. This technique gives an extremely accurate indication of the shape and size of the fetus in early pregnancy and provides the most accurate method of predicting the expected date of delivery (EDD). Because of the relative simplicity, safety, and low cost of the method, and because of the importance of knowing accurately when the baby should be delivered, the ultrasonic scan is becoming almost a routine procedure. It will also detect multiple pregnancy at an early stage and some fetal abnormalities.

The second trimester (13—28 weeks)

Most women are started on iron and folic-acid supplements after booking to prevent anaemia developing later in pregnancy, whilst some authorities also encourage multivitamin supplements and fluoride to reduce the risks of dental decay. A visit to the dentist is advised, and arrangements are made for appointments with the physician every four weeks until 28 weeks. During the second trimester the health visitor will hope to get to know the patient and her family better and be available for help and advice when required. Many women say they have never felt better in their lives than during this stage of pregnancy.

The first movements of the baby, the 'quickening', are usually felt by the mother around 16—20 weeks of pregnancy — earlier in women who have been pregnant before and somewhat later in a first pregnancy.

Problems can arise during the second trimester. Late miscarriages do occur occasionally, when they are more likely to be associated with *cervical incompetence,* a condition in which the neck of the uterus (cervix) opens up prematurely and a premature birth occurs. This is preventable in subsequent pregnancies by applying a purse-string stitch to the cervix, remembering of course to remove it at the beginning of labour!

There are many minor irritations which can cause discomfort and anxiety during pregnancy. A list of some of the more common problems is shown in Table 3.4.

Table 3.4 Minor problems of pregnancy

Problem	Time of occurrence	Cause	Treatment
Vaginal discharge	Any time	May be thrush.	Pessaries and cream.
Backache	20 weeks onwards	Posture, softening of ligaments.	Rest, pain-killing drugs.
Indigestion	20 weeks onwards	Regurgitation of acid.	Antacid tablets or medicine.
Constipation	Any time	Decreased action of bowels.	Diet or a mild laxative.
Poor sleep	30 weeks onwards	Discomfort on lying flat.	Change of posture; possibly tablets.
Leg cramps	30 weeks onwards	Said to be due to lack of calcium.	Calcium tablets.
Stretch marks	30 weeks onwards	Stretching of skin and fat.	None effective.
Chloasma	Any time	Pigmentation of skin, especially face.	None.
Odd aches and pains	Any time	Usually muscular.	Rest.
Varicose veins	20 weeks onwards	Increased pressure in abdomen.	Support stockings or tights.
Piles	20 weeks onwards	Increased pressure in abdomen.	Avoidance of constipation; suppositories or cream.

The third trimester (28—40 weeks)

At this stage of pregnancy preparation for the birth and subsequent care of the baby assume greater importance and many patients find attendance at educational and relaxation classes beneficial, enabling them to understand what will happen later. This is the time to discuss whether to breast feed and some of the advantages and disadvantages are shown in Table 3.5.

The physician and the midwife will probably wish to see the patient every two weeks from 28—36 weeks and will pay particular attention to the size and position of the baby. If the baby seems to be smaller than the dates would suggest then the possibility of inadequate nutrition of the baby due to *placental insufficiency* arises and further investigation may be required. If the uterus seems larger than the dates would suggest then *multiple pregnancy* or an *excess of amniotic fluid*, 'the waters', must be excluded. After 32 weeks it is important to decide if the baby is the right way up — i.e. head down — or whether it is presenting as a *breech* — i.e. bottom first. Most obstetricians would try to turn the baby into the normal position between 32 and 36 weeks.

Table 3.5 Breast feeding

Advantages	*Disadvantages*
Free*	Less freedom for mother.
No equipment	Father cannot help with feeding.
No preparation	May not know if baby getting enough
Milk at right temperature	milk.
Milk contains no dangerous germs	Loose bowel motions means more
Easy when travelling	nappies to clean.
Contraceptive effect	Social embarrassment.
Less risk of breast cancer in	Sore nipple, swollen breast, or breast
mother	abscess may develop.
Closer mother/baby relationship?	Drugs mother taking can pass via milk
	into the baby.
Breast-fed babies compared with bottle-fed babies have less:	
Allergies	BREAST FEEDING IS VERY MUCH
Gastroenteritis	TO THE ADVANTAGE OF THE
Cot deaths	BABY, THOUGH PERHAPS LESS SO
Colds, bronchitis, pneumonia	TO THE MOTHER.
Constipation	
Tooth decay	
Obesity	

*Although no food needs to be bought for the baby, the mother will need extra food while breast feeding.

Haemorrhage

Any bleeding in pregnancy is significant and in the third trimester it is known as antepartum haemorrhage (APH). If it is painless it is likely to be due to a condition known as *placenta praevia*, in which the placenta is attached abnormally low down in the uterus. This condition can be demonstrated by an ultrasonic scan or special X-rays and requires expert supervision by the obstetrician. Bleeding associated with pain in the uterus is more likely to occur from a normally situated placenta which has become partially detached and this condition is known as *accidental haemorrhage*. Again supervision by a specialist is required.

Tests

Most physicians will take another blood test at 30 weeks to check for *anaemia* and for the presence of *antibodies* in *Rhesus-negative* women, and almost all check for these conditions at 36 weeks. This is also the time at which it is usual to assess the size of the pelvis by a vaginal examination, especially in primigravidae, i.e. women having their first baby. The baby's head should go down into the pelvis at this stage and potential problems of *disproportion*, in which the baby is likely to be too large for the mother's pelvis, may be foreseen. From 32 weeks onwards the attendant can usually hear the fetal heartbeat through a stethoscope.

Toxaemia of pregnancy (PET)

In the last four weeks of pregnancy it is usual to see the patient at least once a week to make sure that all is progressing well. It is at this time that *toxaemia of pregnancy* is most likely to occur. This condition is characterized by excessive weight gain — normally a woman should gain no more than 12.7 kg (28 lb) during pregnancy and not more than 0.45 kg (1 lb) per week in the third trimester — by a rise in the blood pressure, and by finding protein in the urine. Slight swelling of the ankles is common in late pregnancy, especially in hot weather, but marked swelling — especially if the fingers and the face are also affected — is often part of toxaemia.

The cause of the condition is unknown but treatment consists of rest and sedation, in hospital if necessary, with induction of labour if the problem persists and the baby is mature enough. The rather strange name *pre-eclamptic toxaemia* (PET) was coined because it has been known for many years that if the condition is not treated appropriately a few patients may go on to eclampsia. In *eclampsia* recurrent fits occur and there is grave danger to the life and health of both mother and baby. Fortunately such an event is extremely rare nowadays provided the antenatal care is good. The management of PET is rest and induction of labour if the condition does not improve. There are no after effects after the birth of the child.

Induction of labour
There are few other indications for *induction of labour or delivery by caesarean section before term* but these may include diabetes or heart disease in the mother or anxiety about the baby's ability to survive in the uterus without risk of danger or death. However, some patients will pass their EDD with no signs of labour and there is some difference of opinion about when and if labour should be induced on the grounds of post-maturity alone. Most British obstetricians would be prepared to wait until at least 41 weeks, provided that the EDD was accurately known, before recommending induction, and some would wait up to another week if there were no complicating factors. However, there is a slightly increased risk of the baby dying in the uterus before delivery after 41 weeks and a considerable risk after 42 weeks so few would delay beyond that point.

If induction of labour is required it may be accomplished by surgically rupturing the membranes — 'breaking the waters' — and the administration of an intravenous drip containing a uterine stimulant. However, it is becoming more common nowadays to administer a new drug called prostaglandin either by mouth or by inserting a vaginal pessary. In either case labour will usually start within a few hours.

Labour

In most women there is no indication to induce labour artificially and the process will commence spontaneously. It is usual to divide the process of labour into three stages. The *first stage* lasts until the neck of the cervix is completely open, the *second stage* until the baby is delivered, and the *third stage* until the placenta (afterbirth) has been expelled.

The first stage

Labour may begin in any one of three ways. The most dramatic is when the *membranes suddenly rupture* and the amniotic fluid drains from the vagina. This can happen without any warning and constitutes the main hazard in attending social events in the last few weeks of pregnancy! Alternatively, there may be a 'show' of *mucus mixed with a little blood* which occurs when the neck of the uterus starts to dilate and the plug which blocks it during pregnancy is released. In either of these cases it is time to prepare for delivery.

Most commonly, however, labour begins when the *irregular contractions*, which have usually become more definite and frequent towards the end of pregnancy, settle into a regular rhythm and become more powerful and noticeable. At this stage it is best to continue to be up and about, to complete last-minute preparations, and to inform any friends or relatives who are likely to be affected. The physician or midwife will advise when it is necessary to go into hospital.

The *length of the first stage* may vary, lasting from an hour or two in some women to 24 hours or more in others. First labours usually last a good deal longer than subsequent ones. The strength of the contractions can also vary enormously but, in general, this increases until the end of the first stage. *Relief of pain* is achieved by relaxation, moral support, and encouragement; the presence of the father is a great help to most women at this time. Traditionally, the use of an anaesthetic machine containing a gaseous mixture (Entonox) of nitrous oxide and air, which the patient can administer herself, and the injection of a powerful pain-killing drug such as pethidine have been the mainstays of treatment during labour.

However, in recent years, *epidural anaesthesia* has become much more widely available. This technique consists of the anaesthetist introducing a small catheter (tube) into the lower end of the spine and injecting a local anaesthetic continuously during labour. This effectively blocks the transmission of painful impulses up the spinal cord and can provide total relief from pain. Unfortunately, some patients dislike the sensation of numbness of the whole lower half of the body which is produced and it is more common for the obstetrician to have to use forceps to deliver the baby, since the normal reflex — which causes the mother to use her voluntary muscles to push the baby out — is abolished.

During the first stage of labour the doctor and midwife check on the progress by listening to the baby's heart, feeling the strength of the contractions, and by examining the mother internally to make sure the neck of the womb is dilating properly and the baby's head is descending through the pelvis as it should. In some units more sophisticated electronic devices will be used to monitor these functions continuously and, of course, if there are any special risks to the baby then extra care will be taken.

In the unlikely event of an emergency occurring during the first stage then the only method of delivering the baby is by *caesarean section.** This consists of anaesthetizing the mother and making an incision through the abdominal wall and the uterus. Between 2% and 10% of babies are delivered in this way, depending on the particular problem encountered and the views of the obstetrician. It is now a very safe procedure for both mother and baby.

The second stage

When this begins the mother feels a strong urge to push and expel the baby. This process may take anything from a minute or two in a woman who has had several children to an hour or more with a first baby. At this stage the physician or midwife will be in constant attendance to monitor progress and to intervene if necessary. The most common and minor form of intervention is to make an incision of the skin under local anaesthetic to enlarge the outer opening of the vagina to help the baby out and prevent damage to the mother. This procedure is called *episiotomy*. It may also be necessary to assist the delivery by pulling the baby out head first by applying *obstetric forceps* or a *suction device* to the baby's head. It is important not to allow the second stage of labour to last too long, since the mother may become exhausted and the baby may be injured. Nevertheless, in most cases *no intervention is required* and the baby can be delivered without intervention.

Naturally, if the presentation is abnormal — for instance if the baby's bottom is coming first, '*a breech presentation*', or if there are *twins*, or if the mother has an *abnormal pelvis* — then intervention is more likely to be needed.

*'Caesarean' because Julius Caesar is reputed to have been born in this way.

The third stage

Once the baby has been delivered safely, the cord is cut, mucus is removed from the baby's nose and mouth to clear the air passages and he or she is wrapped in a blanket to keep him or her warm. It is considered important to give the baby to the mother as soon as possible so that an immediate *bond* may be established and many authorities recommend suckling immediately, since this is said to encourage contraction of the uterus. If father is present as well this should be a moment of supreme happiness for the whole family. The tradition of whisking the baby away for bathing, weighing, and examination has rightly been relegated to a later time.

The mother is usually given an injection immediately after the baby is born to make the uterus contract hard and expel the placenta or afterbirth. The use of this drug, ergometrine, has reduced the usual length of the third stage to less than five minutes and, more importantly, has reduced the risk of post-partum haemorrhage (PPH) occurring before the placenta is delivered. Once the afterbirth has been delivered everyone can relax, an episiotomy can be repaired under local anaesthetic, and the mother can be left to rest. Rarely, the placenta may not be expelled naturally and it may be necessary for the mother to be anaesthetized so that it can be removed manually.

The puerperium

This is the period after delivery, when the mother can recover from the stress of labour and learn to look after her baby and establish a lifelong bond between them. Rather arbitrarily, it is usually considered to last 10—14 days. There is a good deal of controversy about where this period should be spent, although economics seem to be dictating that the time spent in hospital is becoming progressively shorter. This may well be a good thing, since risks to the mother are negligible within a few hours after delivery and the baby — if normal and healthy — will manage perfectly well at home provided the circumstances at home are reasonable. Indeed, many would feel that the development of a close mother—child relationship and the satisfactory establishment of feeding is much more likely to be accomplished in the familiar setting of home and family rather than in the clinical environment of a hospital ward. Even when medical needs dictate a longer hospital stay, (if, for instance, the baby is premature or otherwise at risk) it is most important that the emotional needs of mother and baby should not be ignored amid the pressing technological requirements of modern, intensive paediatric care.

During the puerperium the obstetrician or midwife will keep a check on the mother's progress to be sure that the uterus is diminishing in size, bleeding is minimal, and there are no signs of infection. If the mother had decided against breast feeding then instruction will be provided about the preparation of artificial feeds. It is no longer the practice to give hormone injections or tablets to prevent lactation, since there was some doubt whether these were effective and an increased risk of thrombosis occurring in the leg or pelvic veins after delivery. Early activity is encouraged, since this hastens the return of the mother's body to normal, but she will need a few days' rest from the routine household chores, and the time and opportunity to get used to the new baby. It is most important, however, that other children in the family are not neglected and they should be prepared in advance for the new baby's arrival and encouraged to regard it as 'their' baby, a new addition to the family, and not 'mummy's baby' and thus a threat to their own love, affection, and position in the family (see also Chapter 4).

The mother is encouraged to exercise her muscles after delivery, particularly those of the abdominal wall and the pelvic floor, to improve her figure and prevent later prolapse or urinary problems. Sexual relations may be resumed as soon as inclination dictates and any scars are healed. Contraceptive precautions should be used from the beginning, since conception may occur very soon after delivery. Gradually the family life will return to normal, although if it is a first baby the change in relationships, experience, and lifestyle will inevitably be profound.

The postnatal examination

This is normally recommended *about six weeks* after delivery. It is an opportunity to review the pregnancy and labour, identify any problems or difficulties, and discuss their significance in any future pregnancy. It is also an opportunity to check on any physical or psychological conditions identified during pregnancy and arrange for any further tests or investigations which may be required.

The physician will usually check the blood pressure and weight and examine the patient's breasts and abdomen. An internal examination will make sure that any scars have healed satisfactorily and that the pelvic organs have returned to normal. It is also an opportunity to take a cervical smear to screen for early cancer of the cervix.

Finally, the postnatal examination gives the mother a chance to raise any anxieties or problems she may have and it possibly provides a final opportunity to discuss contraception and help to achieve the object of 'every child being a wanted child'.

4
The new baby

The new-born baby may seem frail and helpless but in fact is remarkably resilient and adaptable. He is dependent on his mother for food and warmth but has well-developed ways of making his needs known to her. The baby feeds when hungry, sleeps when needing to, and cries when uncomfortable. During the later stages of pregnancy, the baby has built up stores of vitamins and iron and obtained from his mother antibodies which render immunity to several infectious diseases. The baby has the capacity to thrive in a wide variety of circumstances and methods of care.

However, the new-born baby is vulnerable in certain important respects, which must be recognized if he is to thrive. In particular the baby must be kept warm, fed correctly, provided with emotional security, and protected from infection.

Objectives of neonatal care

The foundations of the child's future life — physical, emotional and intellectual — are laid in early infancy. Feeding and bowel habits, sleep pattern, emotional stability and many aspects of personality, and the ability to learn and form relationships may be influenced by what happens during the first few weeks.

The objectives of neonatal care must be to produce a happy, healthy infant capable of growth in all these areas, and of resisting physical and emotional stresses.

These objectives are most easily achieved by mature, stable, healthy parents over 20 years old, living in harmony in satisfactory conditions with a baby whom they both welcome. It helps to have family and friends in easy reach. Professional help may be useful, even essential at times, but it is usually of secondary importance.

Table 4.1   Who does what

Midwife	A nurse specially trained for maternity work. Checks progress of mother and baby daily and is on call 24 hours a day for mothers at home. Watches for problems and helps mother establish feeding. Hands over to the health visitor on about the tenth day.
Health visitor	A nurse with additional training in prevention, with special emphasis on the care of young children. May meet parents during pregnancy and after taking over from midwife will visit at home at regular intervals to check baby's development and advise on immunization. Runs the local baby clinic. Available for advice on all aspects of child care, including management of minor ailments.
Hospital paediatrician	Checks baby for abnormalities before leaves hospital.
Family physician	Backs up midwife and health visitor and provides continuing care for baby and family.

Who does what?

Midwife

The midwife is a nurse who has had general training and additional training, experience, and qualifications in maternity work. The midwife, in the British NHS, is in close contact with mother and child once they come home — usually on the second day. She checks the daily progress of both on home visits and is on the watch for problems. She helps the mother to establish feeding and works closely with the family physician and with the health visitor, to whom she hands over care on about the tenth day.

Health visitor (public health nurse)

Also a nurse with basic general training plus extensive additional experience and qualifications covering a wide field, with special emphasis on the care of young children.

She may meet the parents during pregnancy and will home visit during the second week after the midwife hands over and at intervals thereafter to observe the baby's progress and provide any advice or information the mother needs. She is available for advice on all aspects of child care, including the management of minor ailments. She is in charge of a baby clinic held locally to which the mother may go for advice and for the baby to be weighed and checked for normal development.

Physician

While in hospital the baby will be examined by a hospital paediatrician. Once home, the family physician takes over. Each physician has his or her own arrangements for carrying out regular child care and supervision. In Britain this tends to be organized at special sessions, together with the health visitor attached to the practice.

Well-baby clinics

These are usually organized by a health visitor (public health nurse) and held at the family practice or health centre. In addition the physician will arrange to see the children at regular intervals to assess development.

Clinics offer parents an opportunity to discuss any anxieties they may have, to learn what services are available, and to meet other parents and children.

There is no convincing evidence that routine medical examinations of well babies increase early diagnosis of minor abnormalities to the benefit of children. However, it is important for vision and hearing to be checked.

Programme of good care

At birth

The baby should be held by the mother and put to the breast as soon as possible. He will obtain little if any nourishment, but close contact is an important first step in establishing a bond between mother and child and the production of milk is stimulated by the child's sucking. Putting the baby to the breast also causes the uterus to contract so that it returns to its non-pregnant size more quickly. After a short cuddle with his mother, the baby will be weighed, measured, examined by the paediatrician, and left to rest in a warm place.

During the first week

The mother and child begin to know each other and to build up a feeding pattern. He will need five or six feeds every 24 hours at first, as the digestive processes can deal with only small quantities. This has the advantages of frequently bringing the baby close to his mother and of stimulating the production of breast milk. The baby's weight usually falls during this time as he is not taking in enough food to keep pace with his needs and is living partly on his own very adequate food stores. This is normal and should not cause anxiety. It is a mistake to press the baby to take more food than he wants as the digestive tract can cope with only limited amounts. Gradually, the intake increases and most babies regain their birth weight by the age of two weeks.

During the first week a blood test is taken by a heel prick to exclude phenylketonuria. This is an extremely rare, inherited, biochemical defect (it affects only about 1 in 10 000 babies), which is worth checking for because it is devastating in its effects, causing brain damage, and because it responds, if detected early enough, to comparatively simple diets that avoid any complications.

Between eight days and two weeks and again at about six weeks

The baby should be assessed again by the family physician to check progress.

During the first six weeks

It is sometimes difficult, especially for an inexperienced mother, to tell whether her baby is taking enough milk. The actual intake cannot be measured at all if the baby is breast fed, and even a bottle-fed baby may need more or less than average. It is therefore useful to weigh the baby every one or two weeks at first to check that he or she is gaining weight. Later it is easier to tell if the baby is well and growing and frequent weighing is unnecessary.

Common disorders

Cold

A new-born baby very easily becomes chilled and should be placed in a warm room. It does not help to wrap up a cold baby in lots of clothes as he may not be able to raise the temperature inside the bundle because of immaturity. Care must be taken not to burn the baby with a hot water bottle or heater, nor to place a heater where it could cause a fire.

Sticky umbilicus

The cord usually separates by about the eight day leaving a small raw area which, until it heals, may become wet or sticky. It can be treated with surgical spirit and sterile powder. If it has a discharge of pus, or is red or swollen, it is probably infected and the physician should be consulted.

Sticky eyes

In an infant, the tear duct, which drains normal tears from the eyes to the nose, leads from the inner corner of the eye to the back of the nose, is very small in calibre, and easily becomes blocked. The tears, which are constantly being produced to lubricate the eye, cannot then run away and the eye waters and may become sticky. This may be treated by wiping with clean cotton wool dipped in cooled, boiled water. A discharge of pus indicates infection and antibiotic eye drops may be needed.

Hernia

In a small baby a hernia (see Figure 4.1) is caused by a gap between the layers of muscle under the skin of the abdomen. Hernia may occur in the groins, at the umbilicus, and in the midline between the umbilicus and lower end of the sternum (breast brone), all of which are areas where the layers of muscle meet or overlap. A hernia appears as a soft bulge which can be pushed back when the baby is lying quietly but which reappears when he moves or cries.

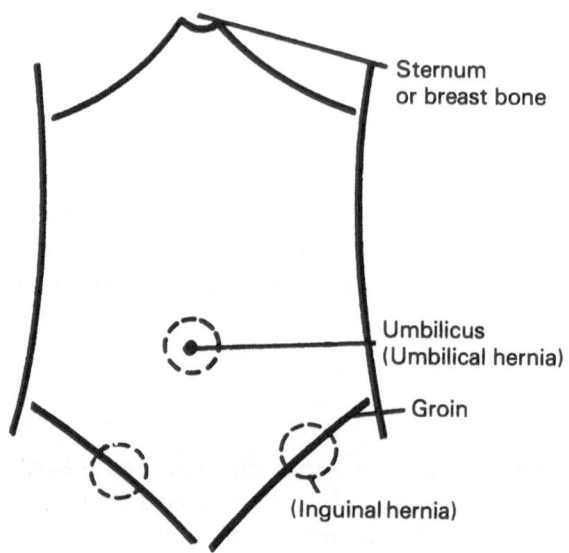

Figure 4.1   Common sites of hernia in a new-born baby.

An umbilical hernia
This is likely to disappear as the child grows and the muscles strengthen and come closer together. This may happen at any time up to 5 years old and an operation to close the gap in the muscles need not be contemplated until after that age. Strapping is not necessary and may delay spontaneous resolution of the hernia by inhibiting the natural movement of the muscles. If an umbilical hernia is still present in a toddler, it bulges when he stands and may seem to be worse than before. This is due to the way in which he stands and not due to an increase in the hernia itself.

An inguinal hernia
This (in the groin) may form a bulge which extends into the scrotum on

the affected side. It is less likely to disappear spontaneously and may require operation to remove the redundant tissue and strengthen the muscles.

Table 4.2   Range of normal

Birth weight	At full term (40 weeks) should be between 2.5 and 4.3 kg (5.5 and 9.5 lb). May need special care if above or below this.
Weight gain	Average 113—227 g (4—8 oz) per week but may be erratic with 340 g (12 oz) one week and none the next. Less-rapid gain in breast-fed babies.
Food requirements	Approximately 2—3 oz (57—85 g) milk for each 0.45 kg (1 lb) of body weight per 24 hours divided between five or six feeds.
Bowels	First stool after birth is dark green or black and sticky (meconium). Changes to brown, then yellow, within 3—4 days. *Breast fed* — soft stools at variable intervals (one at each feed to once a week may be normal). *Bottle fed* — more-formed stools once or twice a day. If baby is well and stools are moist, soft, and pale yellow the frequency of stools does not matter. Should not be persistently green or frothy or contain mucus or blood.
Crying	Normal when baby is hungry, uncomfortable, frightened, or unhappy.
Sleep	Allow opportunity to sleep after each feed, but provided well and contented, amount of sleep does not matter at all.
Head shape	There may be a soft swelling or elongation of the head from pressure as baby came through birth canal. Resolves with time.
Skin	Premature babies are covered with a thick, cheesy substance called 'vernix', while those born late may have wrinkled, flaky skin with long nails.

A hydrocoele

This is a collection of fluid in the scrotum around the testis. It may be present on one or both sides. It is quite harmless, has no complications, and nearly always disappears spontaneously, although this may take several years to happen.

Problems and symptoms

Range of normal

See Table 4.2.

Birth weight

Most full-term babies weigh between 2.5 and 4.3 kg (5.5 and 9.5 lb). Outside this range, the baby may need special care.

Food requirements

Between 57—85 g (2—3 oz) milk for each 0.45 kg (1 lb) of body weight in each 24 hours, divided between five or six feeds.

Bowels

The first stool is normally passed within 24 hours and is dark green or black and sticky. This is called meconium and is the substance occupying the lumen of the bowel during fetal life. As milk passes through the bowel after the first few feeds, the meconium is replaced by the end products of milk digestion and the stools change to brown and then to yellow within 3—4 days. Breast-fed babies produce loose stools at variable intervals; anything from once at each feed to once a week may be normal. Bottle-fed babies usually have more formed stools once or twice a day. If the baby is well and the stools are moist and soft and pale yellow, the frequency with which they are passed does not matter. The stools should not be green or frothy or contain mucus or blood (see page 81).

Weight gain

The average range is 113—227 g (4—8 oz) a week but this may be reached erratically, for instance with gains of 340 g (12 oz) one week and none the next.

Crying

It is normal for a baby to cry when hungry, uncomfortable, frightened, or unhappy (see page 77).

Sleep

This is infinitely variable. An infant should be given the opportunity to sleep after each feed but if he is well and contented, it does not matter at all how much he sleeps (see page 78).

Table 4.3 Normal abnormalities

Jaundice	Yellowing of the skin is normal if it appears on or after the second day and fades completely within five days.
Breast enlargement	Swelling of one or both of baby's breasts. Hormonal in origin and resolves spontaneously.
Vaginal bleeding	Common in baby girls at about the fourth day. Due to withdrawal of mother's oestrogens and requires no treatment.
Purpura of face	A fine purple rash round the eyes from congestion of the face during delivery. Fades quickly.
Bruising	Of face and head after forceps delivery. Soon fades.
Facial rash	Small red spots with yellow heads mainly around the nose. May be treated with calamine. Soon resolves.
Napkin rash	Caused by contact of skin with urine and stool, producing redness of the napkin area, possibly with blisters and weeping. May become very angry, painful, and bleed. Will be cured by: 1 Leaving napkins off altogether whenever possible. 2 Using no plastic pants while rash present. 3 Changing nappy as soon as wet or soiled. 4 Washing bottom with plain water and applying a bland cream like zinc and castor oil each time. 5 Applying nappy like a kilt so it does not lie between the legs.

Head shape

During its passage through the birth canal, the baby's head may be moulded so that it is elongated and pointed at the crown. There is often a soft swelling overlying that part of the head which came first.

Skin

Premature babies are covered with a thick, cheesy substance called vernix. Those born late may have wrinkled, flaky skin and long finger nails.

Normal abnormalities in babies

See Table 4.3.

Jaundice

This is a yellow coloration of the skin causd by the deposition of bile substances from the bloodstream. Normally it appears on or after the second day and fades completely within five days. It occurs because the liver in the newborn cannot cope with the increased turnover of bile products during the first few days of life. It soon catches up and the jaundice fades. Jaundice may develop on the first day of life, if there is rhesus factor blood incompatability. This should be unusual now as rhesus-negative mothers receive an injection after their first pregnancy to prevent the development of rhesus antibodies. Jaundice which persists after the end of the first week in a full-term baby may be a sign of obstruction of the biliary tubes and requires investigation.

Breast enlargement

In the baby, this consists of swelling of one or both breasts. It is caused by a spill over of the mother's hormones into the baby's bloodstream before birth. It resolves spontaneously.

Vaginal bleeding

This is common in baby girls on about the fourth day. It is also probably caused by hormone changes (in this case, of oestrogen) in the new-born. It requires no treatment and is unimportant.

Purpura of face

A fine purple rash around the eyes is common immediately after birth. It is caused by congestion of the face during delivery when small amounts of blood escape from the capillaries into the skin under increased pressure. It has no serious significance, requires no treatment, and fades quickly.

Bruising of the face and head

This may occur after forceps delivery. It soon fades.

Facial rash

Small, red spots with yellow heads — especially around the nose — are caused by obstruction of ducts in the skin with sticky secretion. They need no treatment but calamine lotion can be applied.

Napkin rash

This is a redness of the skin normally covered by a napkin; the skin is sometimes blistered and weeping, and may become angry, painful, and bleed. It is caused by the contact of skin with urine and stool. Ammonia is formed by the interaction of bacteria in the stools and urea in the urine, which causes a chemical irritation of the skin. The inflamed and broken skin may then become infected with bacteria or fungi, such as thrush. The problem is made more difficult by alkaline stools that can occur in a bottle-fed baby on a diet high in fats. Napkin rash is less of a problem in breast-fed babies, who have acid stools. It can be cured rapidly by leaving napkins off altogether. Plastic pants do not cause the original rash but certainly make it worse and delay healing by preventing urine from soaking away, by softening the skin, and by preventing the mother from noticing that the baby needs changing so that wet and dirty napkins are left on longer than they otherwise would be. Plastic pants should not be used at all once a napkin rash is present. The napkin should be changed as soon as it is wet or soiled. Washing with plain water and the application of bland barrier cream, like zinc and castor oil, are soothing and may protect the skin to some extent from the effects of stool and urine. It may be helpful to apply the napkin like a kilt with pins at waist and hem so that it does not lie between the legs. It is unusual for the condition to fail to respond to these measures but if the amount of inflammation is severe and if it persists then antibiotic or antifungal ointments may be necessary.

Infant feeding

Objectives

It is most important for the baby that the mother is as happy and relaxed as possible. If breast feeding comes easily to her and she can do it happily, then it is better for the baby than bottle feeding. If breast feeding makes her miserable, tense, and anxious, then it is better to bottle feed. Whichever method is used, the baby should, as far as possible, be fed when hungry and allowed to take as much as he or she wants. Bottle-fed babies can be as healthy and happy as those who are breast fed, provided they receive the same amount of care and attention. A decision to bottle feed should in no way be looked on as a failure in maternal care.

Breast feeding

Milk is not secreted until the second or third day after birth, and although the baby should be put to the breast during this time, he or she should not be allowed to suck for more than 2—3 minutes on each side or the nipples will become sore. Once the milk is being produced, it is stimulated to flow by the closeness of the baby and by his sucking. The flow can be inhibited by anxiety in the mother. The amount of milk produced depends upon how much the baby takes. Breast milk appears watery in comparison with cows' milk and is sometimes mistakenly thought to be less nourishing or 'not good enough'. In fact it is more suitable for human babies than cows' milk. Overfeeding is impossible in breast-fed babies.

Insufficient milk

This is a common problem during the early weeks, especially if the mother is worried, tired, or unwell or if the baby has been off his or her food and then suddenly regains an appetite. The problem is usually easy to recognize:

The breasts fail to fill.
The baby cries after a few minutes at each breast; demands a further feed a short time later; has small, infrequent stools like firm, green pellets; and fails to gain weight.

The supply of milk will soon recover if the following general principles are followed:

Feeding takes place in as relaxed an atmosphere as possible.

The baby is put to each breast at every feed, care being taken not to let him or her continue sucking once the breast is empty.

A complementary feed is made up beforehand and given after the breast feed if necessary.

The breasts are completely emptied by hand expression after the baby has been fed.

Engorged breasts

The breasts become very tense and painful. If the milk flows when the baby sucks, then this may resolve the problem, but if the milk will not flow, because the ducts are blocked, allowing the baby to suck merely makes the nipples sore. A mechanical breast pump may help. Professional advice should be sought.

Breast abscess

This arises when one part of a breast fails to empty during feeding and bacteria enter through a cracked nipple. The area becomes hard and tender and the skin overlying it flushed. The engorged area may become infected by bacteria. An antibiotic may be required to control the infection. It is quite safe to allow the baby to suck from the affected breast, using it first at each feed, unless the condition is severe or far advanced, when the baby should be fed on the other breast only and hand expression or a mechanical pump used.

Cracked nipples

This is a very painful condition in which the skin of the nipple becomes sore and split. It makes breast feeding difficult, at least for a time. It should be possible to avoid cracked nipples by making sure that the baby does not make the nipples sore by sucking when the breast is empty and by resting the breast for 24 hours, if the nipple is sore, the milk being expressed by hand or breast pump and given in a bottle.

Weaning from the breast

The breast produces as much milk as the baby takes so that the amount available always corresponds to the infant's needs. If less milk is taken, less is produced so that weaning causes no problems if it is done gradually, either by shortening feeds, giving only one breast at each feed or by giving the breast at alternate feeds.

Bottle feeding

Milk for infant feeding is prepared from cows' milk modified to resemble breast milk. A baby cannot digest ordinary cows' milk. The milk has to be specially modified to meet the baby's needs. It is important that the manufacturer's instructions for making up the feeds are followed carefully. It is especially dangerous to make up feeds with too little water as this may cause electrolyte imbalance and too high a level of salt in the bloodstream.

Which milk?

There are no significant differences between brands of artificial milk and therefore no point in changing from one brand to another if feeding problems arise. To do so may simply delay solution of the problem.

How much?

A breast-fed baby takes different amounts at each feed and a bottle-fed baby should be allowed to do the same. Most babies will take what they need and refuse or regurgitate the rest. Some will continue to feed as long as there is milk in the bottle and these have to be rationed according to their weight gain if they are not to become overweight.

How to feed

One of the major advantages to the baby of breast feeding is the close maternal contact. This should be imitated as far as possible for the bottle-fed baby. There is no reason why his father should not also share the feeding but it is best that not too many persons do so.

The baby must always be fed by someone. It is dangerous, as well as disturbing to the child, for him to be fed by propping the bottle up.

Supplements to diet

It is usual to add vitamins A, C, and D to the diet of breast-fed babies and to bottle-fed babies if they are not already added to the powder by the manufacturer. If vitamin C is given in the form of fruit juice, this should not be boiled as the vitamin is destroyed by heat. An excess of vitamins A and D may be harmful so the dose on the container should not be exceeded. Premature babies should be given iron as well as vitamins because they do not have the iron stores which are laid down in the liver of a full-term infant during the later part of pregnancy.

Crying

Crying is an infant's only way of expressing distress. All babies cry when hungry, uncomfortable, in pain, frightened, or unhappy. The degree of sensitivity to these stresses varies from one child to another and for any individual may be different at different times. Even babies have their own personalities — inherited from one or other side of the family. Some children are placid and rarely cry, while others are easily irritated. Some have good and bad periods. Such variations can bewilder parents. It is clear that the variations between individuals to some extent reflect inborn personality traits but it is likely that an infant's environment is a more important factor. The most important factor in the environment is the people around the child, especially the mother. A new baby is acutely sensitive to his mother's state of mind. If she is calm and confident, the baby's vulnerability to stress is low and he cries little. If she is anxious or tense, the baby reflects this in his behaviour, crying for little or no apparent reason, clearly feeling insecure and irritable. A baby's behaviour is a mirror of the mother's state of mind and temperament.

Whether the baby cries or not may depend not only on the intensity of the stress, for instance hunger, but also on the presence of other stresses at the same time. A baby who is cold or lonely will cry sooner, when hungry, than one who is warm and being cuddled or played with. The baby who is anxious and insecure has an ever-present extra stress to make him more vulnerable to anything else which comes along. This situation is a difficult one for parents. All mothers feel anxious to some extent, especially with a first baby; and the more a baby cries, the more anxious the mother becomes. The knowledge that her state of mind is a factor in making the baby unhappy makes her more anxious still and adds feelings of guilt to her more general worries. It is important for parents to recognize this situation, if it arises, partly because understanding what is happening should help them to worry less about the baby's physical well-being and partly because it is impossible to do anything about the vicious circle unless they are aware of it. What action they take will depend on their circumstances but family and friends can help by sharing the care of the child, and the health visitor and physician may be able to reassure the parents that the child is physically well.

It is important for the mother to attend to her own emotional needs in the knowledge that to do so will benefit her baby. She needs adult company, apart from her husband, and interests beyond the domestic routine. However much she loves her baby, he is likely to be dull company and frustrating to be with continuously.

A baby should never be left to cry. Crying is a sign of distress and need for comfort. If his cries are not answered, the baby becomes frightened and a sense of insecurity grows. The distress increases and the baby cries with greater intensity than ever. If the baby seems to be crying to gain attention, then it should be recognized that a need for attention is as important as a need for food. If it is always generously available, then the baby will feel more secure and need to cry for it less.

Sleep

The amount of sleep needed by different children varies enormously. No guidelines can be laid down as to minimum requirements. If a child is happy and well and growing, then the amount of sleep is irrelevant. If the baby is taking less sleep than he needs, this may be a symptom of some other problem, such as abdominal discomfort or anxiety, but it is not in itself harmful. Many new-born infants do not distinguish between night and day and wake for food and attention at intervals throughout both. Some seem to have a reversed rhythm and sleep for a single long stretch during the day and are wakeful at night. This situation rapidly corrects itself after a few weeks. There is no place for the use of sedatives in a new-born baby.

Vomiting

New babies often vomit mucus and liquor swallowed during birth. A summary of the causes of vomiting is shown in Table 4.4.

Table 4.4   Causes of vomiting

Posseting	Most babies regurgitate (posset) a small amount of milk after a feed. May be copious and frequent but baby continues to gain weight steadily and has normal stools.
Overfeeding	A common cause of vomiting in bottle-fed babies.
Unsuitable teat	Milk flows too fast if hole too big and if hole too small then baby may swallow a lot of air.
Poor feeding technique	Air may be swallowed if teat not kept full of milk. Milk will not flow freely unless air is allowed into the bottle to fill the vacuum which develops when baby sucks.
Air swallowing	Caused by prolonged crying, sucking on an empty breast or teat problems.
Intestinal obstruction	A section of bowel fails to develop and so is blocked. Causes vomiting of all feeds from an early age and the passage of meconium is not followed by passage of normal stools (no milk getting through). Rare but important as can often be corrected by an operation to remove the affected segment and join up the normal bowel.
Infections	Any infection severe enough to make a baby ill may cause him to vomit. In addition to vomiting he will appear weak, limp, pale, and off his feeds. Rarely may be from meningitis.
Pyloric stenosis	This results from overdevelopment of the muscle at the lower end of the stomach which then prevents milk from passing into the intestine. Causes violent projectile vomiting during or after feeds in a baby who remains eager to feed but fails to gain weight and becomes increasingly constipated. Commonest in first-born boys, it usually starts in the second or third week of life and is cured by a simple operation.

Minor causes of vomiting

Posseting
Most babies regurgitate, or posset (derived from the word used to describe a drink of curdled milk) a small amount of milk after a feed. The stools remain normal and weight gain continues steadily. This is not true vomiting, although it may sometimes be copious and frequent.

Overfeeding
This is a common cause of vomiting in bottle-fed babies. Little effort is needed on the baby's part to obtain milk and some will guzzle as long as the milk pours from the bottle. An inexperienced mother may interpret her baby's cry of loneliness or discomfort as one of hunger and give him or her an extra feed which is not needed. These situations do not arise with breast feeding as the milk is not so quickly or profusely available.

Unsuitable teat
The milk flows too fast if the hole in the teat is too large. If the hole is too small, the baby may swallow air in an attempt to get milk.

Poor feeding technique
Air may be swallowed if the teat is not kept full of milk. Milk will not flow freely if air is not allowed into the bottle to fill the vacuum which develops when the baby sucks.

Air swallowing
Air swallowing is caused by prolonged crying, sucking on an empty breast, a small hole in the teat, a bottle with a partial vacuum in it, or a teat full of air.

Persistent vomiting, other than possetting, should always be taken seriously, especially if the baby is otherwise unwell, because of the (admittedly unlikely) possibility of a cause needing urgent treatment.

Serious causes of vomiting

Intestinal obstruction
This is due to intestinal atresia. In this condition, a section of the bowel fails to develop so that the lumen, or passage, from mouth to anus is

not continuous. It is rare but important to recognize, as it can sometimes be corrected by an operation to remove the affected segment and join up the normal bowel. It always causes vomiting of all feeds from an early stage. The passage of meconium is not followed by normal stools which prove that milk has traversed the whole gut.

Infections

Any infection severe enough to make a baby ill may cause vomiting. In addition to the vomiting, the baby will appear weak, limp, pale, and off his feeds. The commonest causes are ear, throat, chest, and urinary infections; the most serious is meningitis.

Pyloric stenosis

This results from hypertrophy (overdevelopment) of the muscle at the pylorus (lower end of the stomach). It prevents milk from passing through the pylorus into the intestine beyond. It causes violent, projectile vomiting during or after feeds, usually starting during the second or third week of life. The stools become infrequent and like pellets. The baby fails to gain weight. It is commoner in boys than girls. See Figure 4.2.

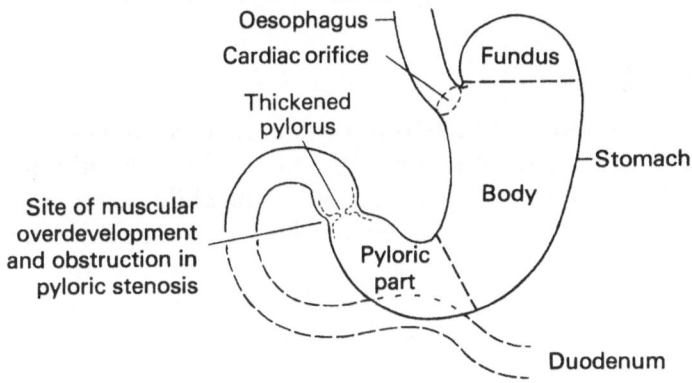

Figure 4.2 Pyloric stenosis.

Bowels

Constipation

This is the infrequent passage of hard stools. It matters only if it causes the baby pain, which is unusual, but it may be a useful sign of underfeeding or the need for more fluids. The breast-fed baby who has his or her bowels open once a week but produces a soft stool is not 'constipated'; on the other hand, a baby who produces a hard stool on alternate days is. In very young infants constipation may be caused by underfeeding or making feeds up with too little water. In hot weather, or if the baby has a fever, it may be because of loss of fluid. Drinks of water may be needed between feeds.

Extra sugar should not be added to the feeds of a constipated baby as it may cause looser stools and lead the mother to believe the problem has been solved. It also causes obesity and induces the child to favour sweet foods.

Diarrhoea

The frequent passage of abnormally loose stools. It should not be confused with the normally loose stools of a healthy breast-fed baby. It is important only as a sign of some other problem or if the baby is ill. In a very young baby it is most likely to be due to overfeeding, incorrectly mixed feeds, the addition of sugar to feeds, or to excessive fruit juice. Diarrhoea, like vomiting, often affects a baby who is ill from some other cause — for instance, an ear infection.

Gastroenteritis

This is an infection of the gastrointestinal tract causing diarrhoea and vomiting. It is now uncommon in the new born in highly developed countries but should be borne in mind if the child seems unwell and especially if there is vomiting as well as diarrhoea. The stools are loose, green, and offensive, and in severe cases, watery with blood and mucus. A breast-fed baby should be allowed to continue to feed but if the baby is bottle fed, milk should be stopped and replaced by clear fluids. The reason for this is that the curd irritates the bowel and the level of salt in the bloodstream may rise when the infant is losing excessive fluid in the vomitus and loose stools. Gastroenteritis is dangerous in infants under six months as they rapidly become dehydrated through loss of fluid. In countries where gastroenteritis is common, special spoons are available to measure salt and sugar to add to boiled water to make up an appropriate solution. The risk of contracting the disease can be lessened by breast feeding and by scrupulous attention to hygiene. In such countries, nothing should be given to an infant apart from breast milk and a sterile vitamin preparation. If gastroenteritis is suspected in a new-born infant, medical advice should be sought. Medicines do not help. The passage of blood either alone or with the stool may be a sign of a serious condition and should be reported, urgently if the baby is ill or in pain.

Colic

This is an intermittent abdominal pain occurring in spasms repeated at variable intervals. Intestinal colic is caused by violent contractions of segments of the intestine which interrupt the normal, gentle, rippling waves of muscular contraction which are called peristalsis. It makes the baby scream (different from the hunger cry) and draw the legs up. In infants it can be caused by taking feeds too fast, overfeeding, swallowing air, too much fruit juice, and by anxiety.

It is not clear whether 'three months' or 'evening' colic is really due to colicky abdominal pain. It affects babies under three months old and is associated with screaming after feeds, especially during the evening. It is worse in first babies and when the mother is anxious and may respond to a change in routine, the father taking over the evening feed or playing with the baby for a while after it. It may help for the couple to study the reasons for the mother's anxiety, especially her exhaustion at the end of the day, and work at ways of resolving these problems. She may have to be less houseproud, let her husband prepare the evening meal, or make other adjustments to her routine.

Skin

Milk rash

This term is often used to describe the small, pink spots with white heads which affect many infants around the nose and across the cheeks. It is not clear what causes them but they have nothing to do with milk and should be left alone.

Neonatal acne

This looks like, and may in fact be, a severe form of milk rash. The face becomes red with lumpy spots containing what looks like pus. They should not be squeezed. Calamine lotion may be used. It clears spontaneously but if it is severe and worrying the parents, then it should be discussed with a physician.

Infections

Skin infections in new-born babies may cause blisters or redness and swelling of the skin, especially around the umbilicus and nails. They are caused by bacteria invading the skin. They can be potentially serious and medical advice should be sought. Proprietary antiseptic creams are best avoided as they can cause sensitivity reactions and the inflamed skin is more susceptible than ever to bacteria.

Convulsions

The human brain responds to strong irritants such as poisons or high fever by discharging massive electrical impulses which cause a convulsion. The brain of a child is more sensitive than that of an adult and in about 6% of children a convulsion can be caused by a level of fever commonly encountered in childhood illnesses. This does not mean the child has epilepsy. It merely indicates that at that time, he or she has a low threshold of brain irritability. The baby loses consciousness, goes stiff, and may roll the eyes, grunt, make grimaces, clench the fists, or twitch. A convulsion is most likely to be caused by a high fever from an infection such as tonsillitis but rarely it is caused by meningitis or another serious condition, so medical advice should be sought.

Most convulsions are very short and are over before help arrives. It therefore does not matter if the physician is not there within a few minutes. He is needed more to decide what to do next than to treat the convulsion.

While waiting for the physician to arrive, the baby should be laid on his side, so that no vomit can be inhaled, undressed, and cooled with a cloth wrung out in cold water.

5

Pre-school and early school years

Children's health

Children are much more healthy than ever before. That is true if we measure health as less risk of dying and more freedom from major illnesses.

A look at Figure 5.1 shows that mortality in childhood has fallen markedly and that many fewer children suffer from major illnesses such as tuberculosis, poliomyelitis, mastoid infection, and rheumatic fever.

However, the mass of sickness in childhood is no less in volume — but is much less dangerous and much less severe.

No fewer children suffer from common colds, earaches, sore throats, gastric and intestinal disturbances, bed wetting, eczema and asthma, and nervous problems.

Figure 5.2 is the overall morbidity over 30 years in children and it shows little change. Children still are becoming sick and parents and doctors still have much to do — but the worries over complications and permanent after effects are much less, because there are fewer serious ill effects. Parents and physicians must apply commonsense management for the common ills of children, realizing that many of them are inevitable accompaniments of growing up.

Both must be concerned also with applying preventive measures to try and prevent problems and diseases. This consists not only of a

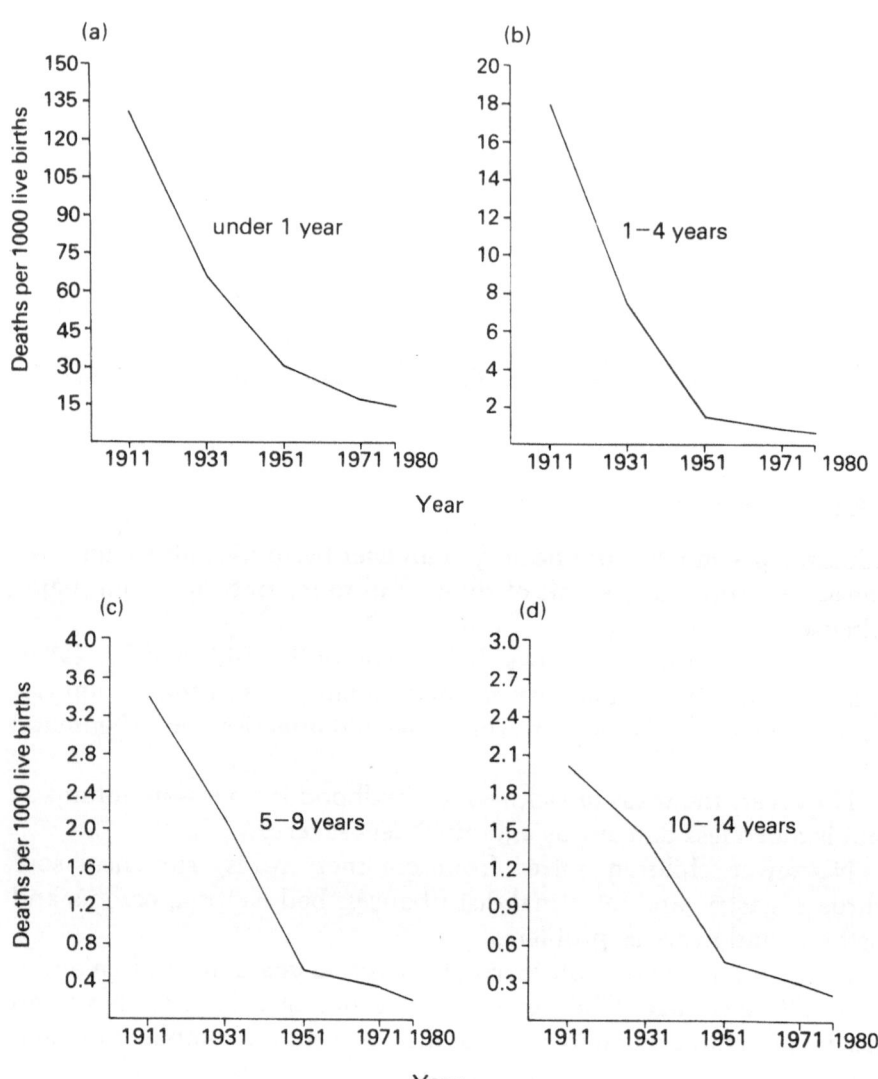

Figure 5.1   Childhood mortality (a) under 1 year (b) 1—4 years (c) 5—9 years
(d) 10—14 years.

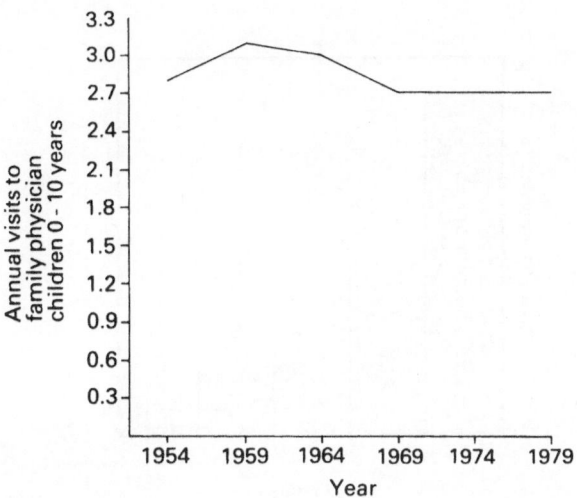

Figure 5.2   Childhood morbidity in a general practice, 1950–1980.

series of immunizations aimed at preventing childhood infections but also of laying down foundations for a healthy adult life avoiding unhealthy, hazardous habits. It must include a sensitive and a sensible system of parenthood through which children can be taught the rules of health, disease, and accident prevention as well as the rules of good and decent human behaviour.

Common causes of ill health

The most common causes of ill health are infections of the respiratory tract — the nose, throat, ears and chest; skin rashes and spots, of which allergies, eczema, boils, and similar infections are more common; gastric and intestinal infections with sickness and diarrhoea and tummy aches of various causes; the common infections such as chicken pox, mumps, measles, and whooping cough (the last two should be preventable by injections) and german measles (rubella) (which should be prevented in subsequent pregnancy by immunizing girls aged 12–13 years); accidents, which are the greatest cause of death in children after the first year; and problems of behaviour and the emotions (Figure 5.3). The major dramatic diseases such as

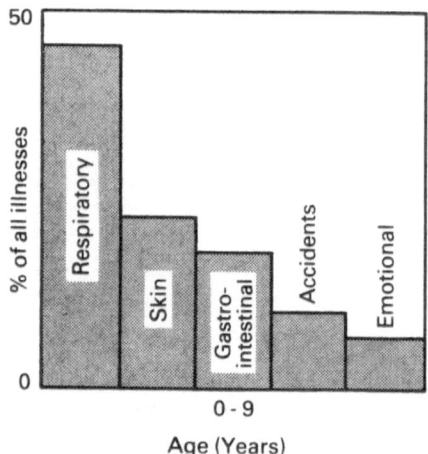

Figure 5.3   Common diseases in childhood.

leukaemia and cancer, meningitis, arthritis, fibrocystic disease and coeliac disease, and mental disease are rare. They cause great worry and distress to families who are unfortunate enough to have such problems but their incidence must be kept in a proper perspective.

To provide such a perspective it may be useful to give approximate numbers of new cases of such major diseases in a typical average family practice of 2500 persons compared with other more common disorders that a family physician can expect to manage in any year (Table 5.1).

Table 5.1   Incidence of children's illnesses (1—10 years) in a family practice of 2500 persons (300 children under 10) per year

Minor illness	No. per year
Coughs, colds, and catarrh	200
Skin rashes and spots	75
Vomiting, diarrhoea, or abdominal pains	60
Earache	60
Sore throat and tonsillitis	50
Chickenpox, mumps, measles, etc.	30
Accidents	30
Bed wetting (at age of 7)	10

Table 5.1 Continued

Major illness	
Bronchitis or pneumonia	25
Asthma	5
Epilepsy or convulsions	3
Appendicitis	1
Leukaemia and cancer	1 new case every 10 years
Mongolism	1 new case every 10 years
Spastic	1 new case every 15 years

To recap the *most common illnesses of children* are:

Infections of the respiratory system
    Coughs, colds, and catarrh
    Croup (laryngitis)
    Earache
    Sore throat
    Wheezy chests

Skin rashes and spots
    Allergies (urticaria or nettle rash)
    Eczema
    Warts

Infections and upsets of stomach and intestines
    Vomiting and diarrhoea
    Tummy aches

Specific fevers and infections
    Chickenpox, mumps, etc.
    Flu and similar viruses

Accidents

Ingredients for good health

There are no secret or magical measures that will ensure good health in childhood.

The *basic ingredients* are to provide the right mix of sound family care, social environment, educational and play opportunities, and freedom and encouragement for each child to grow and develop at his or her own rate.

The *family* has to provide the child with loving care and support to create a feeling of belonging to a close and protective caring unit that gives shelter, clothing, food, and other necessities.

The *local social environment* has to provide friends and playmates and places to play, explore, imagine, and daydream in safety and with stimulation.

The *school* must be more than a teaching factory. It must provide the setting for learning more than the 3 R's. It has to help to develop personal character and behaviour, to detect learning and developmental difficulties, and to try to remedy these in close collaboration with parents.

Children basically have very healthy and tough bodies that have to adjust physically and emotionally to a hostile environment. Physically they have to learn how to avoid accident hazards at home, at school, and on the road. They have to build up their own natural immunity to foreign organisms, such as viruses and bacteria, assisted by artificial immunization when available. It is inevitable that their immature and 'virgin-white' bodies will suffer respiratory, gastrointestinal and skin infections from foreign hostile organisms until they establish a tougher maturity and resistance.

A programme for preventive care

The commonsense approach must be to take whatever measures are available for specific prevention such as immunization; following the rules of the road when walking, running, playing, and cycling; and avoiding other known hazards through dirt and unhygienic habits.

Life and living are a risky business and nothing can be perfect. Prevention can never be complete and hazards can never be completely avoided. Parental over-protection may be worse than a certain amount of positive wilful neglect. It is difficult for parents to avoid self-blame when accidents happen and diseases occur, but most are unavoidable and no one is to blame.

There is no uniform static programme for effective preventive care. There is no evidence that regular check-ups in children are any more effective than they are for adults. In themselves they do nothing to promote health or prevent disease.

Certainly there should be a close relationship with the physician responsible for the child's care and there should be no barriers to seeking his or her help and advice when parents need it.

Apart from immunization at the appropriate time there is no evidence that tonics, vitamins, or other supplements improve health in normal children of normal families eating a normal diet.

Immunization

Killer disease like diphtheria, tetanus, whooping cough and so on are far less common and less virulent than at the turn of the century. The main reasons for this are social ones with increased resistance to disease coming from better food and better housing with less over-crowding and probably also from a change in the character of the germs themselves.

Vaccination has also played its part in the decline of these diseases but has a far more important role to play in preventing their return. For the germs are still in the community and are ready to attack non-immunized people.

During the first years of life children are particularly vulnerable to infectious diseases. Indeed infections are still the commonest cause of death in the first year of life and the second commonest (after accidents and violence) in 1—14-year-olds.

A baby has some immunity from his mother which lasts about 3—4 months. After that he has to develop his own. This can be achieved either by catching infections and surviving them or by being vaccinated against them.

Vaccination means using germs that have been killed or modified to be very mild to make the baby produce immunity without suffering the bad effects of the disease. Unfortunately not all vaccinations are completely free from side-effects or risks although they are all far less dangerous than catching the diseases they prevent.

For a few children the risks of vaccination against some diseases are higher than normal (see Table 5.2) and therefore vaccination should be avoided. For the large majority the risks of disease far outweigh the risks of vaccination and it is vital that they complete as full a programme as possible (see Table 5.3).

Table 5.2 Reasons for not being vaccinated

Vaccination	Contraindications
Diphtheria	None
Tetanus	None
Whooping cough	History of fits in the child or family history of fits. Any abnormality of the brain or nervous system. An acute illness with a fever (wait until better then vaccinate). Severe reaction to a previous dose of vaccine (no more whooping cough but continue with others).
Polio	An acute illness with a temperature ⎫ wait until ⎬ better then Diarrhoea and/or vomiting. ⎭ vaccinate Allergy to Penicillin and some other antibiotics. Radiotherapy, cancer drug therapy, steroid therapy. Cancer. PREGNANCY.
Measles	As for polio. History of fits in the child or family history of fits. Allergy to eggs. Active TB.
B.C.G.	As for polio (except allergy to Penicillin). Septic skin conditions. Chronic skin disease e.g. eczema.
Rubella	As for polio. Pregnancy and any possibility of pregnancy within 3 months of vaccination.
Influenza	Should not be given to any child below age 9 years. As for polio (except allergy to antibiotics).

N.B. If your child suffers from any serious illness or you have any doubts about a vaccination then consult your doctor BEFORE any vaccination is carried out.

One argument some parents put forward against immunization is that their child might not catch a particular disease and therefore any risk from vaccination is too much. This does not really stand scrutiny as, for example, by the age of 14 about 90% of non-immunized children will have caught measles and 70% will have caught whooping cough and chickenpox. Those that haven't and catch infectious

Table 5.3 Possible schedule of immunization (for UK)

Immunization	Age of child
Diphtheria ⎫	⎧ 3 months
Whooping cough ⎬ 'Triple'	⎨ 5 months
Tetanus ⎭	⎩ 11 months
(mumps usually included in USA)	
Poliomyelitis	⎧ 3 months ⎨ 5 months ⎩ 11 months
Measles	14 months
Diphtheria ⎫	
Tetanus ⎬	4–5 years
Poliomyelitis ⎭	
Rubella (German measles)	11–12 years (girls)
BCG (tuberculosis)	13 years

diseases when they are older may often have more serious illness and complications.

Let us now consider vaccinations individually.

Polio

Use of the vaccine has virtually eliminated the disease. There is a risk of paralysis in about 1 in 4 million children vaccinated and any non-immunized parent or sibling should be vaccinated at the same time as the child.

Whooping cough

This is undoubtedly the vaccination which worries most parents. Since the concern over its safety was first voiced in 1974 the percentage of children, under 2 years, vaccinated has dropped from 78% to 38% and there has been a major rise in the incidence of whooping cough (102 000 cases in 1977—79 epidemic).

Facts about which there is little argument include:

Whooping cough remains a serious disease causing death (28 in 1977—79) as well as an unknown number of cases of brain and lung damage.

10% of children below the age of 2 with whooping cough have to be admitted to hospital.

Medical treatment is unsatisfactory.

Vaccination is over 90% effective.

Minor reactions to vaccination (irritability, temperature, sore arm, vomiting) occur in up to 10% and resolve within 24—48 hours.

Facts about which there is some argument include:

Whether or not the vaccine causes fits — 6—9% of children will have a fit in childhood so fits are common at the age the vaccine is given. For many children the vaccine may cause their first fever and this may provoke the fit rather than the vaccine directly. There is no test which proves that fits are due to the vaccine and indeed there is some evidence that they are not.

What the risk of brain damage from vaccination is — The vaccine does seem to cause some cases of serious brain damage. A recent massive investigation has shown that if all the 600 000 (normal) children born in Britain each year undergo a full course of vaccination with whooping cough vaccine then six will have a severe reaction and be left with a permanent disability. 75% of cases developing serious reactions to the vaccine will have done so within 24 hours.

Avoiding vaccination if a child suffers from any of the conditions shown in Table 5.2 will lessen the risk of brain damage.

For normal children the benefits of whooping cough vaccination outweigh the risks though only you, the parents, can decide for your children. The Department of Health strongly recommends the vaccination and all the authors' children have been vaccinated against whooping cough.

Measles

Measles remains a highly infectious disease which can be serious in young children.

Vaccination is over 90% effective and in about 5—10% of children will produce symptoms of mild measles 6—12 days after being given. It can produce a febrile fit in about 2 per 1000 children (7 per 1000 from measles itself) and encephalitis — infection of the brain — in about 1 in 100 000 (1 in 1000 from measles itself).

Tetanus

A course of 3 injections gives complete protection for at least 5 years. There are no ill effects.

Vaccination at the time of an injury where tetanus is a risk is unsatisfactory as protection will not develop in time to deal with any possible infection from that wound.

BCG

Between the ages of 11 and 13 all children have a test to see if they are immune to TB. If not they are given BCG vaccination. Any baby who is going to come into contact with any person who has had TB in the past should also be vaccinated.

Rubella

Vaccination may be followed by mild fever, rash, cough, arthritis in 10—28 days. Protection may decline 5 or more years after vaccination.

Any woman planning to have a baby who is not certain that she is immune to rubella should have a blood test done and be vaccinated if necessary.

Children have to catch diseases like colds, sore throats, mumps, chickenpox, and glandular fever if they are going to develop immunity to them. For many of them there is much to be said for catching them in childhood rather than in adulthood when their effects may be more severe.

There is no point in isolating children who are contacts of another child who has an infectious disease. Let them lead their normal life and watch them for the incubation period of the disease (see Table 5.4). If they develop the disease then normally there is no point in isolating them from their brothers and sisters as firstly children are often

Table 5.4   Incubation periods

Disease	Incubation period	Length of time child is infectious
Chickenpox	11—21 days	1 day before to 6 days after start of rash.
Measles	10—15 days	5 days before rash to 5 days after temperature is back to normal.
Mumps	14—21 days	3 days before swelling until swelling goes.
Rubella	14—21 days	5 days before to 4 days after start of rash.
Scarlet fever	2—5 days	21 days or until after 1 day on penicillin.
Whoopingcough	7—10 days	4 days before to 3 weeks after start.

infectious before you know they actually have a disease and secondly it will often be better for the others to catch the disease while they are young. It is advisable to keep children away from adults who may not have had the disease.

Who does what?

All who are concerned with caring for children have certain responsibilities and roles.

Parents

Parents are most important! It is they who provide the stock factors with their transmitted genes and chromosomes and who then add to them with a home and social environment that will influence the child's development.

Parents must take steps to make the best use of available health services, they must know what is necessary, what is available, when, and where.

Parents must be able to provide *self-care* for most minor ailments and problems of children. It is salutary to note that parents can manage three out of four of all childrens' ailments and problems adequately.

The primary health care team
This consists of physician, nurse, and health visitor (public health nurse), who have the roles and the responsibilities to provide readily available and accessible facilities to which parents can bring children for routine preventive and medical care.

It is their function to support, educate, and inform parents as well as to provide more traditional care and cure for children.

Hospitals and specialists
These play an important but small part in the care of a few diseases and problems of children. Less than 10% of all children in any year require care from specialists or hospitals.

Schools and teachers
Children spend more than half their lives at school and the potential influences on their health and development are considerable — ranging from risks of cross-infection from other children, to assisting with emotional and educational development and medical supervision.

Common problems and symptoms

When something is wrong or just not right with a child the first step must be to take note of the presenting symptoms and problems, then to decide what they signify and what needs to be done about them.

This is a logical but a far from easy approach. When adults have symptoms or problems, at least they can put them into words and describe their feelings and sensations as 'symptoms' and a 'medical history' is available from which the physician can begin to make a definitive diagnosis.

With children it is more difficult. They cannot put their feelings clearly and accurately into words. Parents and doctors have to rely on other features from which to decide when a child is unwell, what is wrong, and what to do about it.

How do children 'complain'?

Despite apparent theoretical difficulties, in real life the situations generally are more easy to analyse and resolve. There are a few and limited sets of common symptoms and problems that a child presents:

Slow development or lack of progress.
Behaviour problems.
Altered habits.
Normal abnormalities.
System symptoms.

Slow development or lack of progress
Children follow a certain broad pattern of development. They walk and talk at recognized times. They learn at broadly similar rates. They advance and pass accepted landmarks of development approximately at similar ages.

An apparent delay in the development of one skill may cause anxiety but it has to be realized that there are huge ranges of the normal responses. Walking, talking, manipulative skills, and social habits do not all develop at the same rate. A more justifiable cause for worry is when all stages of development are delayed. Then a detailed professional assessment is necessary.

Behaviour problems
Children are individuals. They inherit characteristics from their parents. They are influenced by their home, school, and environment. They can and do react to stresses and strains by altered behaviour.

They may exhibit fears and terrors which may manifest themselves overtly as tummy aches, nightmares, skin rashes, or wheezy chests, or as fear of school or other manifestations of apparent misbehaviour.

Altered behaviour may occasionally be an early symptom of some underlying physical illness, but this is unusual and sooner or later is accompanied by other symptoms in the child.

Altered habits
Within the spectrum of normal habits such as eating, sleeping, and bowel movements there is a wide range of normal responses. Children do not eat all at the same rate, or with the same gusto, or the same quantity. Their appetites range far and wide and high and low. Poor appetite by itself is not an indicator of illness. Many normal children have periods when they eat less — much less — than their parents believe that they should. Fickle appetites are common and normal in

healthy children. There is no need for extra vitamins, tonics, or other measures.

Sleeping habits vary. Some sleep 12 or more hours soundly every night. Others make do with almost one half this amount. Both are normal. There is no magic or required length of sleep that everyone, children or adults, have to have. Each has his or her own range.

At times sleeping habits may become disturbed because of children's anxieties or fears arising from problems at home or school. Sleep may become disorganized for a period that may extend into weeks or months, but eventually becomes stabilized given time, understanding, and support.

There is no uniform and standard pattern of *bowel movement or consistency*. Constipation is never a disease unless it is the result of obstruction of the intestines; a very rare event in children. There is a range of normal from one bowel movement a week to four each day. Either pattern may be normal in healthy children.

If the motions are hard and evacuation causes pain and distress, then the simplest and safest measure is to increase the bulk of food roughage with bran and bran cereals, fruit and vegetables, and wholemeal breads.

About one in ten of children still *wet their beds* (enuresis) most nights at the age of 5 years, and the proportion is still one in twenty at the age of 10.

Voluntary control of the bladder takes longer to develop in some children than in others. Rarely, it is caused by diseases such as infections or disorders of the nervous system, which can be excluded by a physician.

In itself enuresis is harmless, but it causes great distress to the child and the parents and results in extra costs of bed linen. It always ceases eventually.

There are ways in which the child can be helped — by using behavioural training methods such as alarm bells that ring when the bed becomes wet. This may help to speed up development of automatic bladder control. Most important are general understanding and support by parents and praise for dry nights. The child must never be scolded or punished. He or she (boys are more prone to enuresis) cannot help wetting the bed. As a general rule drugs are not required, but there are a group of tricyclic drugs that sometimes help.

Normal abnormalities

Within the spectrum of normality there is a wide range of responses. Just as some children are taller than other children, so some are thinner and some are plumper. Some are fair and pale and others are dark and ruddy. Some are inclined to knock knees and others to bow legs. Coughs, colds, and catarrh are so prevalent as to be inevitably normal, as are infections such as chicken pox and mumps, and measles and whooping cough unless the child is immunized. It is as well that these infections are caught in childhood and that children develop a life-long immunity, because these infections in adult life produce more severe reactions.

System symptoms

There are some more specific symptoms that are related to body systems. Although these may help in pinpointing the problems, nevertheless it may be often difficult to arrive at an absolutely satisfactory diagnosis and explanation.

Pain generally is an indication of some local disorder. Toothache relates to an infection or exposed nerve. Sore throat and earache too are good specific localizers, but tummy ache and headache are less so.

Pains in the abdomen may signify an acute infection or digestive disturbance or rarely an acute appendicitis. Recurrent bouts of tummy ache, especially in the mornings during school time, are very unlikely to be associated with any active abdominal diseases. It is much more likely that they are due to some anxiety or fear in the child.

Headaches in children are unusual. When they do occur they are unlikely to be due to eye strain, and very rarely are they due to some brain disorder or meningitis. Much the most likely reasons for bouts of headache in children are that they represent a form of migraine or, like tummy aches, may be the outcome of some underlying tension or anxiety.

Children have a labile temperature-regulating mechanism and can run a *high fever* readily. The height of the fever is relatively unimportant. A fever represents the body's natural protective reaction to an infection. It serves a useful purpose in 'burning-up' foreign organisms in the body. Artificial attempts to lower the temperature are rarely necessary, except in children prone to febrile convulsions. It is more important to make an accurate diagnosis of the cause of the fever and then either leave the infection to settle on its own as in influenza, measles, and the common cold, or treat the condition with specific antibiotics, when necessary, as in tonsillitis, middle-ear infections or urinary infections.

The three most common sets of *symptoms of local system disorders* are coughs, cold and catarrh, earache and sore throats; skin rashes and spots; and sickness and diarrhoea.

These are the three systems most exposed to the ill effects of the environment. We breathe continually and we may inhale viruses and bacteria and atmospheric pollutants that lead to coughs, colds, and catarrh. Likewise when eating we may swallow organisms or irritant foods that may cause local irritation with sickness, diarrhoea, and abdominal pains.

The skin offers a huge exposed surface area for external infection or irritation. The skin also may react to ingested or inhaled substances by allergic skin rashes and spots.

Common diseases

The catarrhal child

All children pass through a period, between 3 and 8 years of age, when they are particularly likely to suffer from repeated colds, coughs and catarrh, earaches, sore throats, and wheezy chests.

They are all part of the same basic disorder, linked structurally and causally.

Figure 5.4 shows the anatomical proximity of the various parts.

The explanation of these well-nigh inevitable disorders is that the child's immature breathing system is not able to deal effectively with the many new germs and irritants that are encountered when children first start to mix more widely on playgrounds and at school.

Though a process of increasing natural immunity, resistance is built up gradually over a few years.

Figure 5.5 shows the frequency of these conditions during the first ten years of life with a peak at 3—7 years followed by the natural decline after 7—8.

Most children apparently need to suffer the immunological experiences of a series of these infections to establish their own natural

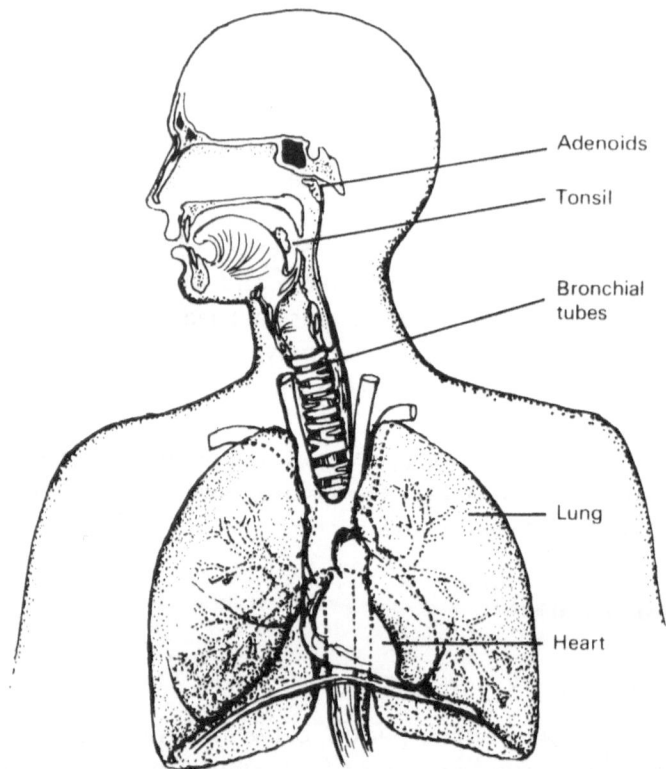

Figure 5.4   Structure of the airways.

resistance — at present there is no way of artificially providing them with immunity. The *causes* of the various conditions that make up the catarrhal child package are varied.

Many viruses and bacteria may be isolated from children with coughs, colds, earache, sore throats, and wheezy chests. There is no single organism that can be blamed. But that is not the whole story. Other factors are important, such as inherited family allergic tendencies and individual proneness to attacks not due to any discernible inherent permanent weakness. Social class does not affect the frequency of these conditions, but certainly their effects are more serious in lower social groups.

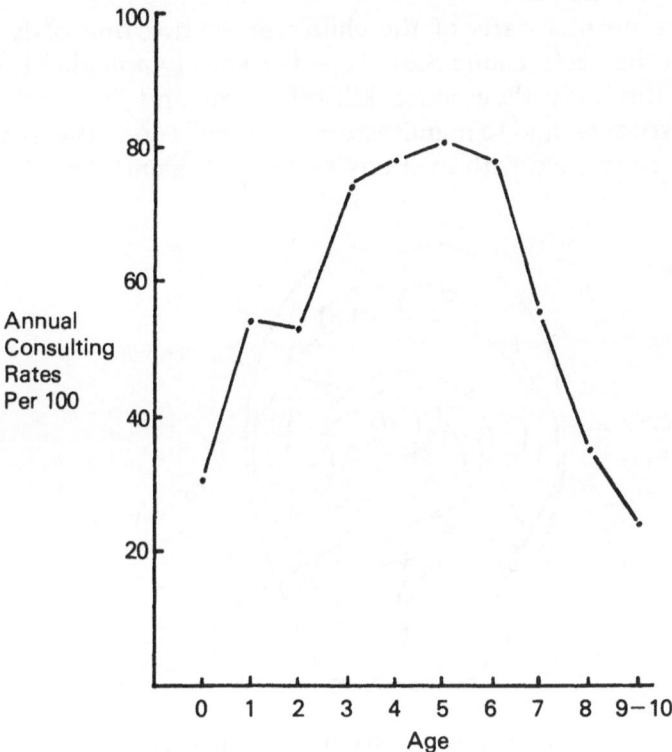

Figure 5.5   Frequency of colds, coughs, catarrh, earache, sore throat, and
wheezy chest.

Coughs, colds, and catarrh (CCC)
All children in the 3—8-year-old age group develop coughs and colds.
They are a normal abnormality. In some a state of persistent catarrh
and nasal obstruction also is normal.

There are no ways of avoiding or preventing them. There are no
effective curative remedies, although relief can be obtained from some
cough mixtures.

Antibiotics, vaccines, vitamins, and other pseudo-specific measures
are useless and unnecessary. Removal of tonsils and adenoids does not
provide a cure-all.

Tonsils and adenoids

These are normal parts of the child's protective ring of lymphatic tissues in the neck (Figure 5.6). Together with lymph glands in other parts of the body they act to kill off germs and deal with foreign inhaled irritants, and to manufacture blood cells and other substances specially concerned with the body's defences against infection.

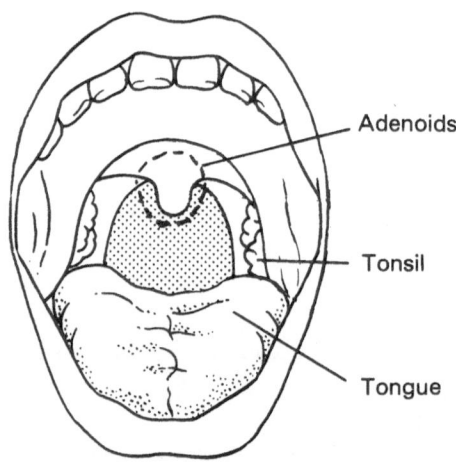

Figure 5.6   Protective lymphatic ring.

All children have relatively large tonsils, adenoids, and neck glands compared with the size of these tissues in adults. They enlarge because they work more in children to deal with the germs that are encountered for the first time. They enlarge because they participate in the immunity-building process by which children build up their natural resistance. They will shrink and become smaller after the age of 9—10 years, once this natural immunity has been created.

Tonsils and adenoids should not be removed just because they appear large or because children have repeated coughs and colds. They are important components of nature's defences.

There are a few reasons for considering removal of tonsils, such as when children suffer from frequent attacks of real tonsillitis. Adenoids may need removal if they cause obstruction to tubes that connect the back of the throat and the ear (the Eustachian or tympanic tube). Such

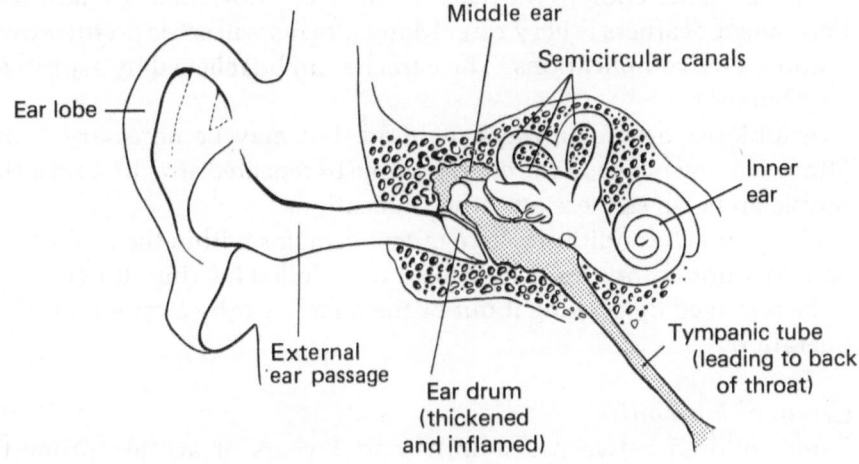

Figure 5.7   Acute otitis media — regions affected.

obstructions may predispose the child to recurring middle-ear infection.

In the 1930s four out of every five children entering high class schools in Britain had had their tonsils removed. Now the rate is one in five — probably still too high. Probably, less than one child in 50 needs to have his or her tonsils and adenoids removed.

Earache

Earache in children is most often due to an infection of the middle ear (*acute otitis media*). It results from spread of infection along the tympanic tube by bacteria or viruses.

The infection leads to inflammation and swelling of the lining of the middle ear with an accummulation of mucus. The child experiences earache. There may be associated fever, vomiting, and general malaise. The accummulated mucus and pus may discharge through the ear drum. The hearing is dulled temporarily.

Acute otitis media is common. More than one half of children suffer one or more attacks. It is now a much less serious condition than 20—30 years ago. The organisms have become less virulent. The general health of children is now much better. Effective treatments are now available (Figure 5.7).

Spread of infection to the mastoid air cells is now almost unknown. Permanent deafness is very rare. Many attacks will settle on their own without any complications. The earache can be relieved by aspirin or paracetamol.

Antibiotics are not always required, but may be necessary if the attack is a severe one, if the child is prone to repeated attacks, and if the physician believes there are other indications.

Glue ear is a condition where mucus remains within the middle ear and does not absorb quickly. This causes dulled hearing. It may need to be removed by sucking it out of the middle ear by a minor surgical operation.

Croup or laryngitis

Some children between 9 months and 3 years of age are prone to laryngitis when they suffer a cold. The infection settles on the larynx producing a characteristic barking cough that is worse during the night.

It is a most frightening experience for the parents to be awakened at night by their child who sounds like a dog or a seal barking and who appears to have some difficulty in breathing.

'Croup' is an old English term for the condition. In days past it was associated with diphtheria. Now all children are immunized against diphtheria and the cause of the croupy cough is a virus.

Although the cough and breathing difficulties are alarming the attacks usually clear in a few hours with warm drinks and a soothing linctus. However, the symptoms may return nightly over 2–3 nights. Admission to hospital is rarely necessary. Antibiotics are not helpful since almost all are caused by viruses which are unresponsive to antibiotics.

Wheezy chests

In some children colds tend to 'go onto their chests', producing wheezing and breathlessness. These children appear to have ultra-sensitive bronchial tubes that over-react to infections by producing too much bronchial mucus, by excessive swelling of their lining and by spasm and tightening of bronchial muscles.

These wheezy attacks do *not* signify that the children will develop asthma in later life.

The attacks respond well to antibiotics and medication to relieve the swelling and spasm of the bronchial tubes.

Gastrointestinal infections and infestations

The second most common infections are those of the *stomach and intestines.*

This is not surprising because eating offers the opportunities for foreign germs and irritants to be swallowed into the stomach. Once swallowed, the stomach and the bowels react by endeavouring to remove the offensive substances by vomiting and/or diarrhoea. Sickness and diarrhoea are common in children. Except in infants they are of no serious significance. The attacks tend to pass in 2—3 days. Medicines and antibiotics are not required. The best management is to omit solid food until the attack passes but to encourage drinks of clear fluids or fruit juices.

Threadworms (pin worms) are common in children. They are harmless apart from causing itching of the bottom that is worse at night.

There are many effective drugs that will destroy the threadworms, but recurrence is common.

Abdominal pain

When a child is unwell for any reason, he or she may complain of a tummy ache — although the cause of the illness may not be within the abdomen. Such tummy aches may be associated with ear or throat infections or with emotional upsets.

Repeated and recurrent complaints of tummy ache may be an expression of emotional disorder. They are common in children when they first start school or when they face other problems. There is rarely an underlying disease within the abdomen and the child's more general problems have to be understood and resolved.

Appendicitis, or other major intra-abdominal disorders, are rare. Appendicitis is not an easy condition to diagnose early even by a physician. Any abdominal pain in a child that persists for more than 3—4 hours and is accompanied by vomiting should be assessed by a physician.

Common skin problems

It may be a surprise to realise that *warts* are the most common skin disorder in children after infections such as boils and impetigo.

Warts are caused by a virus. They occur most often on hands, and on feet (where they are called verrucae). Warts will disappear naturally if left alone. If they are a nuisance they can be treated with various ointments or paints or frozen with liquid nitrogen or carbon dioxide.

Some children have skins that are sensitive to external or internal irritants. *Eczema and urticaria* (nettle-rash) are manifestations of such hypersensitivities. They can be controlled by external applications of steroid creams for eczema and by anti-allergy medication for urticaria.

Genitourinary problems

There are very few medical indications for *circumcision* — but there may be religious reasons. Most little boys do *not* need to be circumcised. The foreskin does not separate completely from the underlying glans penis until the boy is aged 4 or 5 years. It is quite wrong to force back the foreskin — this causes pain, bleeding, laceration, and scarring.

In a few boys their testes may not descend completely into their scrotum (*undescended testes*). All little boys should be examined to ensure that testes have descended by the age of 5—6 years. If not, a minor surgical operation can be carried out to bring them down and tether them into the scrotum. If the testis remains undescended in the groin it is more exposed to injury and disease and may lead to infertility.

Infections of the bladder and kidneys are more common in girls than in boys. They may cause bouts of fever, vomiting, abdominal pains, and bed wetting.

Sometimes the cause may be a congenital malformation of the kidneys, ureters, or bladder. All children who suffer repeated attacks of urinary infections should be investigated by X-rays and other means so that any such defects may be corrected and further attacks prevented.

Fits and convulsions

A small proportion of children suffer from *epileptic fits*, which may be associated with brain damage in a few.

A more common cause of convulsions in young children (6—18 months) is *febrile convulsions*. Some children's nervous systems over-react to high fever by convulsions with shaking, twitching, and temporary loss of consciousness.

Such febrile convulsions rarely lead to epilepsy in later life.

Febrile convulsions tend to last for a few minutes only. They are alarming but are not serious or dangerous in themselves. The child will come round unassisted. Management is aimed at preventing any injuries during the period of unconsciousness and to ensure a free airway.

The attacks are caused by fever, which may be caused by conditions such as otitis media, chest infections, or (very rarely) meningitis. Such underlying infections must be treated as well as the convulsions.

Accidents

Children and old persons are the two groups most prone to accidents.

Some accidents are inevitable and are part of the process of growing up and learning about what is possible, what is safe, and how it should be done.

Many accidents are preventable and it is up to parents, teachers, and others to teach children how to avoid preventable accidents.

The child with a major illness

Unfortunately, a few children will suffer major illnesses that will produce serious handicaps and may even shorten their young lives.

Apart from the help that modern medical and surgical sciences can give and the support that social and nursing services can provide, parents undertake much personal care.

There are no universal hard and fast rules, but certain guidelines may be useful.

As normal a routine as is possible should be followed. The child should go to school, he or she should be allowed and encouraged to participate in normal social and sporting activities, and treated with kindness and understanding but without excessive sorrow or sympathy.

At home a regular routine should be created and followed that encompasses medical, educational, and social needs.

If the child becomes housebound then it is necessary to maintain contact and communication with the outside world through the radio, television, and reading. Friends should be invited and encouraged to play as often as possible. A certain amount of honesty may be valuable, although children do adapt well and approach serious illness with a great deal of optimism and a strong belief in miracles. They often cope better than their parents and if a child is seriously ill then it is very important that the adults affected do not allow themselves to get carried away by the emotions that are inevitably aroused.

Child development

A child's intelligence is largely genetically determined but a good, stimulating, loving home environment is essential to help any child to achieve the best he possibly can.

Increase in size is *growth* and increase in complexity is *development*. Development takes place in different fields (locomotion, manipulation, use of eyes and ears, general understanding, speech, bladder control, etc.) and depends on the maturing of the brain and nervous system and so cannot really be speeded up by outside stimulation. On the other hand, once a baby is ready for further development in a particular area, then stimulation and practice by parents is important.

All babies follow the same sequence of development but the rate of development varies from child to child. Indeed, even the same child does not develop at a constant rate but in lulls and spurts.

Normal children will be faster or slower than average for the activities listed in Tables 5.5 and 5.6 and a normal child may not walk until 17 months, talk until 15 months, or gain bladder control until 2 or 3 years. If a child is slow in only one particular area, then this is not a sign that he is retarded. It may be due to a family trait, e.g. slowness of speech or bladder control may run in the family; or to lack of stimulation in that particular field, e.g. if a child is never allowed to attempt to feed or dress because Mum always does it, then he will be late in learning these skills; or to physical disease, e.g. lateness in speech may be due to deafness.

Only if a child is badly behind in all developmental activities should there be any suspicion that he is retarded or emotionally deprived.

Table 5.5 Some aspects of development to note in first year of life

4 weeks	Watches Mum when she talks to him.
6 weeks	Smiles at Mum. Begins to follow moving persons with eyes.
3 months	Holds rattle placed in hand. Follows object with eyes through half a circle.
4 months	Excited when sees toys. Laughs aloud. Starts to show interest in things. Turns head to a sound.
5 months	Can lie on tummy with weight on forearms. Able to reach for object and get it. Smiles at self in mirror.
6 months	Chews and begins to show likes and dislikes of food. Can be held in standing position taking weight on legs.
7 months	Feeds self with biscuit and can feed well with cup. Responds to name. Says Da, Ba. Transfers objects from one hand to other although most objects end up in mouth.
8 months	Sits unsupported. Leans forward to grasp objects. Responds to "No". May say Da-Da, Ba-Ba.
9 months	Stands holding onto furniture. Trys to stop Mum washing face. Can pick up small object between thumb and forefinger.
10 months	Creeps. Waves bye bye. Helps with dressing. Starts letting go of things deliberately.
11 months	Says 1 word with meaning though understands others. Shows interest in pictures in books.
12 months	May be shy. May kiss if asked to. Says 2—3 words with meaning. Walks with one hand held.

Note 1. If baby is premature then subtract the number of weeks he is premature by from his age to get the age at which his development should be.

2. These are average times for babies' development and normal babies may well be late doing some things. However the later a baby is then the less likely it is to be normal for that area of development. These ages only provide a rough guide.

Table 5.6 Some aspects of development to note in second and third years of life

13/14 months	Walks with no support.
15 months	Creeps upstairs. Keeps throwing things on the floor. Takes off shoes. Feeds self. Can build a tower of 2 bricks.
18 months	Can climb stairs and throw ball without falling. Seats self in a chair. Manages spoon well. Can point to pictures in book and name simple objects. Tells Mum when wants potty. Largely dry by day. Copies Mum doing simple housework. Delights in doing the opposite of what is asked.
21 months	Can pick up object from floor without falling. Knows 4 parts of the body. Obeys simple orders (if wants to). Can ask for things. May have sleeping difficulties.
2 years	Turns pages of books singly. Puts on some clothes. Washes and dries hands. Talks a lot using I, me, you. Dry at night if lifted late in the evening.
2½ years	Jumps on both feet. Can walk on tiptoe. Gives full name. Attends to toilet without help (except for wiping bottom). Still highly negative.
3 years	Dresses and undresses self if given a little help. Joins other children in play. Always asking questions. Begins to draw things.

Please see notes at bottom of Table 5.3

As well as physical and mental development, a growing child is also developing his *personality and character*. The child is an explorer, intent on making new discoveries in all fields of experience. This is how he learns and develops; by exploring the environment by getting as far from base as he can or dares and by poking fingers into every nook and cranny. He touches, looks at, tastes, and smells everything, constantly absorbing information. The child also explores emotionally. He experiments to find new ways of pleasing, and of annoying, the parents. He does awful things just to find out how they will react, and if they react negatively may continue just to find out what will happen next. The child plays with noises and words and ideas and learns that he has an identity separate from his mother. There is a need to experiment with this new-found independence but at the same time a need for the security of knowing that a parent is near and will always provide love. It is only from this secure base that he can make progress and develop a stable personality and a full range of intellectual skills. This combination of dependency and the need to explore and experiment makes a toddler a very difficult person to live with. The child needs to know that he is loved and valued however awful the behaviour and so it is important that parents never let it seem that their love is dependent on good behaviour. They have somehow to be able to show, when necessary, their disapproval while at the same time confirming their love.

Sometimes a child's bad behaviour is a deliberate attempt to gain attention. This is particularly likely to happen if the mother is tired or irritable or busy with a new baby. His need for love and attention are greatest at such times, when the mother is least able to provide them. Being naughty may be the only way to attract her attention. Even if the mother is cross with the child that is better than being ignored, and so he continues to misbehave, and may taunt her by soiling or refusing to eat.

It is easy for a mother to reach the evening and realize that she has not said a kind word to her toddler all day. He may then refuse to go to bed. During the night the child feels frightened and insecure and cries out for her. The next day she is more tired than ever and he is naughtier. It is at times like this, when a child is least lovable, that love is most needed. Only if completely assured of the parents' love and the place in the family can the child develop fully. Parents need not worry about exerting their authority over a child. Good discipline results more from praise and encouragement when good than punishment when naughty.

Children have a very strong natural wish to please their parents. They find that to do so produces a warm, pleasurable response which they enjoy. They have a natural desire to experiment, but behaviour problems such as waking at night, refusing to go to bed, refusal of food, and soiling arise from a feeling of insecurity. This can be resolved only with love and patience. There is no place for punishment.

6
Adolescence

What is it?

Adolescence means literally 'growing up', referring to the period between childhood and manhood or childhood and womanhood. The precise limits of adolescence are difficult to define since the physical and psychological changes in both boys and girls are gradual and take several years to develop fully. However, it would be generally agreed that adolescence normally occurs between the ages of 10 and 17 in girls and a little later on average in boys, perhaps between 11 and 18 years.

Puberty, on the other hand, has a rather more precise meaning since technically it refers to the age at which a young person becomes functionally capable of procreation. Whilst in practice, of course, this is also rather variable, for legal purposes the age of puberty in English law is 12 years for girls and 14 years for boys. *Menarche* is even more precise for the individual girl since this is defined as the age at which the first menstrual period occurs, usually between 10 and 16 years of age.

Girls

The first sign of adolescence in girls is breast development, which precedes the growth of pubic and axillary hair by a year or two and the onset of the menarche by an even longer period. Initial breast develop-

115

ment is often asymmetrical and this can give rise to anxiety in the child or her parents. Tenderness of the developing breast tissue, sometimes termed 'mastitis of puberty', is also common, but is of no significance. It is important to know that boys also may have some swelling and tenderness of one or both breasts at this stage and it is important to reassure them that there is no likelihood that they will change sex!

The processes of adolescence are started by changes in the primary sexual organs, the ovaries and the testes, under the overall control of the pituitary gland at the base of the brain. In girls, the ovaries are stimulated to produce oestrogens and later progestogens and gradually the secretion of these hormones begins to develop into the cyclical pattern which will be present for the rest of a girl's reproductive life.

Because it takes some time for the body to settle into a regular rhythm the early cycles are often anovulatory, i.e. they occur without an egg being released from the ovary. This may be associated with infrequent, irregular, or very scanty periods initially. This is of no consequence but the converse may happen and very frequent or excessively heavy periods may occur which are distressing for the girl and may require medical treatment. Emotionally, the onset of menstruation can be an alarming event for any girl who is ill informed and it would seem appropriate that instruction should be provided by the parent or teacher well in advance. Any embarrassment or difficulties may then be minimized and psychological trauma avoided. Subsequent changes in adolescent girls include the completion of breast development and adult distribution of hair, widening of the pelvis and hips, and a general rounding and feminization of the body contour, often after a period of gawkiness.

Boys

In adolescent boys secretion of testosterone by the testes leads to rapid growth of the genitalia and the development of pubic and axillary hair, together with a growth spurt during which growth in height often outstrips the development of a more muscular adult male body contour. The major change noted socially is the 'breaking of the voice', which occurs when laryngeal growth leads to conversion of the choirboy's piping treble into the adult bass or tenor. Penile erection does not start in adolescence. It is physiologically possible from birth onwards, but it does become more frequent in association with developing sexuality and at this stage masturbation and 'wet dreams', with involuntary emission of semen during sleep, are normal occurrences.

Health and illness

The requirements for maintaining health and avoiding disease in adolescence do not differ greatly from those at other times of life, although the emphasis may be different. A sensible, well-balanced diet with adequate amounts of protein, fibre, and vitamins and a limited amount of fat and carbohydrate is required, but during the growth spurt the adolescent's requirements may be higher than at any other time of life and provided that obesity is avoided a large appetite is not pathological.

Most children at school are required to take part in games and physical training but there is often a hiatus after leaving school when this valuable habit may be lost. Sport can also provide a social outlet and lead to the development of new interests and relationships. For those children with an academic bent the stress of studying for examinations is a major factor in their lives, whilst for those who leave school at 16 or so the stress of starting work with adults in shops, factories, and offices may be considerable. Suitable preparation and support during this period should help to prevent or minimize the emotional strain. When one considers that these major changes in life style are occurring against a background of rapid physical growth and the developing pressures of an awakening sexuality, it is perhaps not surprising that adolescents are particularly vulnerable to behavioural problems such as abuse of alcohol or drugs, unwanted pregnancy, venereal disease, and suicidal gestures. In addition, adolescents are likely to suffer injury from occupational or sporting hazards, whilst road-traffic accidents represent the major risk to life and health.

Who does what?

By far the most important influence in the lives of most adolescents is the quality of *parental care and guidance*. If the parents are able to provide a loving and supportive background, and at the same time can allow the child to develop his or her own personality and gradually become more independent, then the foundations of healthy emotional maturity have been laid.

The *school* has responsibilities over and above its narrow educational function in that horizons may be widened, social functioning improved and support and guidance offered where parental supervision is lacking.

Health visitors (public health nurses) are an important link between the school, where problems are often identified, and the primary health care team. The *family physician* may learn of difficulties occurring and add this to his or her background knowledge of the patient, to be used at some later date when the opportunity arises. He or she remains responsible for providing primary health care for the individual adolescent and for arranging specialist consultation and admission to hospital on the rare occasions when this becomes necessary. If the physician is able to work with a community psychiatric nurse then he or she has an excellent opportunity to intervene positively at an early stage in the emotional and behavioural difficulties of adolescence and prevent the development of self-destructive behaviour patterns.

For some teenagers parents, schools, and doctors all represent unacceptable authority and alternative sources of aid and support should be available. These may be provided via youth centres and special counselling agencies or walk-in facilities where informality is the keynote and help is offered by persons only a little older than the teenagers themselves.

Presentation of symptoms and problems

The most difficult problem for the family physician in his dealings with his adolescent patients is the establishment of an efficient and sensitive relationship. The adolescent may see his or her physician as an authoritarian figure, closely identified with the parents and apt to divulge confidential information to them against his or her wishes. There is no reason why the young person's confidence should not be safeguarded by the same ethical rules that govern any other consultation, so that what passes between the participants during the consultation is private to them. Nevertheless, there are circumstances in which the physician must apply heavy pressure to the adolescent to encourage them to communicate directly with their parents. In most circumstances it is possible to achieve the desired result where it is in the adolescent's interest.

The sensitivity and extreme self-consciousness exhibited by some adolescents is also a potential problem. A girl who has yet to come to terms with her own sexual maturity may be too embarrassed to approach her family physician, sometimes even if the physician is herself a woman. Similarly, there may be a fear of the physician laughing at their apparently trivial worries or just failing to listen to the real problem. In all these circumstances the relationship may be facilitated if the physician has used the opportunities presented during childhood to show that he or she regards the youngster as a person in their own right, separate from the parents, and capable of answering questions, complying with treatment, and generally taking an intelligent interest in their own life and health. By adopting a friendly, understanding, and supportive educational approach the physician can help the young patient to develop a sensible attitude towards health, confidence in self-management of minor illness, and an awareness that he or she can approach the doctor for help with any problem ranging from acne to contraception, or emotional problems to drug abuse.

Diseases of adolescents

Infections

The need for immunization against infectious diseases has largely disappeared by adolescence with one important exception — *rubella*. Rubella or german measles is normally a trivial viral infection, but in early pregnancy the developing fetus may be infected, with catastrophic results. For this reason all adolescent girls should receive rubella vaccine between 11 and 13 years of age, i.e. before they are at risk of conception. Failing this, any adolescent girl should be immunized when the opportunity presents itself so long as pregnancy can be definitely avoided for at least three months. One dose of vaccine usually provides protection for life. A booster dose of tetanus and polio vaccine is also recommended in this age group and, of course, specific immunization against other diseases may be required before travel overseas.

Teenagers are less likely than children to suffer from colds, earache, and chronic catarrh, but they are still prone to *tonsillitis*, which may require antibiotic treatment. One antibiotic which should not be prescribed in these circumstances is ampicillin, since the sore throat may be the first sign of *glandular fever*, a condition which is most prevalent in this age group. If ampicillin is given to anyone incubating glandular fever they are very likely to develop a severe rash all over the body and to feel very unwell. Glandular fever (or infectious mononucleosis) is a virus infection with a slow onset, characterized by sore throat, fever, swollen glands, and sometimes a rash. The diagnosis has to be confirmed by a blood test and there is no specific treatment. Recovery can sometimes take several weeks in a severe case.

Infectious hepatitis or 'yellow jaundice' also occurs in this age group. This is caused by a virus infection of the liver. Again, there is no specific treatment and recovery may be prolonged. Girls commonly suffer from a first attack of 'cystitis'* at this age. This unpleasant condition, caused by infection in the urine, makes the patient pass urine frequently and painfully and is treated by drinking lots of fluid and taking a course of antibiotics. This condition may be precipitated by sexual activity, hence the term 'honeymoon cystitis', but this is by no means the only precipitating factor. Naturally, sexual experience also leads to the risk of sexually transmitted diseases such as *gonorrhoea*. In a boy this causes a discharge and pain on urination but a girl may have no symptoms whatsoever. However, if she has contact with someone who has gonorrhoea she must be investigated and treated to prevent secondary infection of the uterine tubes, leading to infertility later.

Other medical problems

The most common skin problem of adolescents is *acne*. This condition is caused by hormonal changes leading to abnormal secretions of the skin glands. The glands produce an excess of sebum, a greasy substance, which hardens and darkens on contact with the air to

*See Chapter 20.

produce 'blackheads'. These block the ducts and the skin glands swell and become inflamed leading to 'spots', 'blind boils', and sometimes frank boils or abscesses with resultant scarring. Treatment is aimed at encouraging the glands to drain by applying hot, soapy water and gently removing the 'blackheads'. Tetracycline, an antibiotic, may be given by mouth in severe cases and prolonged treatment for several months is usually effective. Exposure to sunlight or an ultraviolet lamp is also of value, but none of the creams, ointments, powders, or other applications have been shown to have any useful long-term effect. Provided scarring can be prevented the adolescent may be reassured that all will be well in the long run. Nevertheless, the psychological distress caused by this disfiguring problem may be very considerable at this age and a sympathetic approach is essential.

Verrucae, or plantar warts, are also a common nuisance and can give rise to considerable pain on walking. They may be painted, soaked, burnt, or frozen off but one must be careful not to leave a tender scar in the foot which will persist forever. Left alone all warts eventually disappear.

Asthma is less common in adolescents than in children but may persist or even present for the first time in this age group. *Hay fever* is more common and can cause a good deal of disability in the summer months, especially at examination time. There is now a wide range of drugs available which can give relief to the sufferer, without producing drowsiness.

Abdominal pain is not an uncommon symptom and may be caused by a great variety of conditions. However, teenagers may be particularly prone to colicky pain arising from an oversensitive bowel, which is sometimes associated with diarrhoea and the passage of slime or mucus. This often requires no treatment but the passage of blood with the motions should always be investigated further. Another type of abdominal pain often first experienced by girls at adolescence is associated with ovulation, when the egg is released from the ovary approximately midway between the menstrual periods. This may be associated with quite a sharp pain in the lower abdomen and may need to be distinguished from some more serious cause of pain such as *appendicitis* or *ectopic pregnancy*.

Much more common is *spastic dysmenorrhoea*, or period pain, which tends to be at its worst on the first day of a period. Most girls experience some pain or discomfort but more severe pain requires rest and a pain-killing drug such as aspirin or paracetomol. In severe cases the contraceptive pill is a highly effective treatment for dysmenorrhoea, although it is not generally recommended until the menstrual cycle is well established. All other forms of contraception (see Chapter 2) are suitable for adolescents, except that the coil or IUD is not generally recommended for girls who have not had a pregnancy. Vaginal discharge and itching due to *thrush* is a common problem in teenage girls and is amenable to treatment with cream and pessaries, plus if necessary the abandonment of tights and nylon pants (see Chapter 2).

Emotional and behavioural disorders

Perhaps the most difficult area of concern is in the field of *emotional and behavioural disorders*. Adolescence is a time of experimentation, of rebellion, and of attempts to find an identity. Inevitably, experimentation with socially acceptable drugs such as *alcohol* and *nicotine* occur and, just as inevitably, some young people will go too far. This is, of course, more likely to happen if they have serious problems of insecurity and no stable home base. *Cannabis* — 'pot' or 'grass' — is quite freely available and many authorities doubt whether it is any more dangerous than cigarettes or alcohol. However, there can be no doubt that experimentation with the 'hard' drugs — for example *heroin, morphine, amphetamines, barbiturates*, and *LSD* — can lead to addiction, degeneration, and sometimes an early death. Any youngster who has risked taking these dangerous substances must be advised to consult his or her physician and should be given a sympathetic hearing if he or she really wants help to break the habit. Unfortunately, it is often parents who consult because they are concerned that their child may be abusing drugs or alcohol. They may have noticed a change in behaviour: staying away from home, unusual irritability, moods of elation interspersed with deep depression, loss of jobs, glazed eyes with pinpoint pupils, bouts of abdominal pain, vomiting, sweats, and trembling. Whilst these symptoms may be present with or without other suspicious circumstances, it is difficult for the physician to make contact with the patient unless he or she accepts help. Not infrequently, the physician has to wait until the young person is convicted by the courts for a drug-related offence before any treatment is possible.

Another aspect of living in a drug-oriented society is the availability of *tranquillizers and antidepressants* which may be taken by teenagers in suicidal gestures. In most of these instances the intention is not to commit suicide but either to provide a brief oblivion and so escape a stressful situation or, more often, to attract attention and sympathy by a so-called 'cry for help'. Inevitably, emotional reactions provoked by parental rejection or failure of a love affair may produce severe crises in adolescence, but the easy availability of drugs must increase the risks of self-poisoning.

Intense interest in religious, political, and other cosmic matters is normal, especially amongst intelligent adolescents, but occasionally the physician may have to differentiate between normal interest in these matters and a degree of interest which may suggest a serious mental abnormality such as early *schizophrenia*. More commonly, adolescents may exhibit marked *anxiety* and *depression* which would have serious implications in an older person but which may disappear within a few days in the emotional volatility of adolescence.

Anorexia nervosa is a condition occurring in this age group, usually in girls and young women. The characteristic feature is an abnormal aversion to food, so that the girl loses weight and becomes weak. Her periods will cease and her secondary sexual characteristics such as breasts and body shape become less feminine. Indeed, some authorities see a psychological explanation for the condition as an attempt to avoid growing up, with all the responsibilities this entails.

Adolescents need help from parents, teachers, physicians, and other professionals and counsellors to develop a realistic view of themselves, their intelligence and capabilities, interests, ambitions, and social and family situation. This requires skilled, non-directive, non-authoritarian, non-invasive counselling, patience, understanding, and a memory of the times when adults were teenagers themselves, with the same adolescent problems.

7

Marriage and family

The quality of a marital relationship and of family life affects the health of all members of the family. Ill health of all sorts, from sore throats to heart disease, is more common in persons under stress, and domestic unhappiness is the commonest source of stress. A happy and secure home seems to provide increased protection against sickness, whilst unhappiness makes everyone more vulnerable. As well as having an immediate affect on health, the quality of family life influences the ability of children to lead healthy lives and form satisfactory relationships when they grow up.

Adults develop most of their attitudes and techniques of living from what they learnt at home in childhood. Their relationships with the opposite sex are based on the models provided by their parents. Their diet, attitudes to smoking, alcohol, and work are all subject to the same powerful influence. Children whose parents are unable to make marriage work are more likely to have serious marital problems. Children of smokers are more likely to smoke. Fat parents tend to produce fat children.

Healthy living

Most modern diseases are the direct result of an unhealthy way of life. A healthy life style contains the following elements:

A nutritious *diet* containing all the essential elements, including roughage, and avoiding excessive animal fats, tea, coffee, or alcohol.

Regular *exercise*.

Avoidance of *cigarette smoking*, *obesity*, and *excessive stress*.

Prevention of disease by *immunization*, e.g. against diphtheria tetanus, polio, whooping cough, measles, and rubella.

Early recognition of treatable disease by medical checks such as blood pressure measurements (every 5 years) and cervical smears (every 3—5 years).

If everyone followed these guidelines, diseases such as lung cancer, heart disease, stroke, and cancer of the cervix would cease to be the scourges of early middle age.

The future health of children depends on their childhood experience.

Family life

If a child is to grow and develop to the full his intellectual and emotional potential, and capacity to learn and make relationships, he needs love, security, and respect from the parents. He needs to be completely certain of their love and to know that it is not conditional on good behaviour or achievements. The mutual respect which develops between a child and the parents in such a relationship means that his desire to please them is ever present and concepts of naughtiness and disobedience do not arise. The parents' expectations are realistic. The child is confident and free from anxiety and all his energy is available for growth, development, and learning.

Parents providing this sort of family life for a child have first to have established a satisfactory relationship for themselves. This has to be based on love, tolerance, and mutual respect; a degree of maturity at marriage is helpful. Couples who are aged under 20 when they marry are more likely to divorce than those who are older.

Most couples have to accept that they cannot each satisfy all the needs of the other: intellectual, social, and sexual. Most marital relationships have to be flexible enough to allow outside activities and friendships even if sexual fidelity is preserved. To love someone is to depend on them, and this applies to parents and children as well as to husbands and wives, but overdependence of one person on another is damaging to the relationship. Each individual has to retain his or her own identity and independence if the relationship is to thrive. This is nearly always easier for men than for women.

Work and marriage

A man is usually expected to have work and interests outside the home; a woman often is not. Even before she has children, a woman's job usually has a low value set on it. Her job is often looked upon as 'helping to pay for setting up home' and as 'giving her something to do while waiting for a family'. She is more likely than her husband to have given up friends and outside interests on marriage and is therefore in danger of becoming socially isolated, intellectually frustrated, and overdependent on both husband and children. It benefits everyone in the family if she can maintain her own independence and self-respect.

Starting a family — when and why?

Couples now can usually plan whether and when to start a pregnancy. It is important that care is taken in making this decision. It is too often taken for granted, even by the couple themselves, that they will have children. However, in one in ten marriages one or both partners are sterile. The marriage needs to be well established and stable and they should decide to have a baby only because they want one and not because they think it will 'bring them together' or because family, friends, or society expect it of them. Everyone should at least consider the option of not having children.

The spacing of children should also be the subject of the same careful consideration. The traditional pattern of having a second child when the first is 2 years old was established before contraception was generally available. It is not necessarily the best interval for every family.

A happy, secure 4-year-old welcomes a new baby with unreserved pleasure. He is sure of his parents' love and approval and understands explanations and abstract ideas of time, such as: 'I will play with you when I have finished bathing the baby'. He joins in caring for the baby. The elder child's position in the family is well established and he can do special things with the parents from which the baby is excluded. He is toilet trained and well settled at a nursery school or play group. Self-confidence and an ability to express adequately enable him to be proud of the baby.

The 2-year-old has none of these advantages and often suffers as a result of the division of his or her parents' attentions. He constantly has to be restrained and is well aware that no one ever grumbles at the baby. The more the child loves the baby, the harder it is for him to bear any resentment. As the child grows older and goes to school, he plays with children of the same age. The 2-year gap is too large for close companionship. Some families make the 2-year gap work very well but a longer one is worthy of serious consideration.

Problems within marriage

Despite the best endeavours of the partners, marriages sometimes break down. It cannot be denied that this is always traumatic and damaging for the children of the marriage, but with care and thought the damage can be minimized.

The main problems for the children are coping with feelings of rejection ('if Daddy had loved me enough he would not have left me'); of guilt ('if I had been good, Daddy would have stayed'); of anger against one or both parents and maintaining love and respect for both parents. With immense self-control, it is possible for parents themselves to help children with these emotional turmoils. They need to be encouraged to express their feelings and to be shown that they are understandable and not wicked. They need to be reassured that both parents still love them and thought carefully about them before deciding to separate, that it seemed the best thing for everyone, that the one who has left is not a bad person, that it was not the fault of the children that the marriage broke down. If the bitterness between the parents is too great for this, someone else should attempt it. The best person may be the court welfare officer, a relation or friend of the family, social worker, teacher, priest, or any one of a number of people.

Sometimes the greatest strains on a marriage occur when the

children reach adolescence. This is the time when it is especially important for the woman to have maintained her own independence, self-respect, friends, and outside interests. As the children grow up and need her less, she is likely to feel rejected and useless. Her husband may not be able to fulfil all her needs. If she is overdependent on either him or her children, the relationships will suffer. If she can avoid this, allow the children to stand on their own feet, be an interesting companion as well as a loving, tolerant wife and mother, the members of the family are more likely to maintain close links for the rest of their lives.

8
Middle age

What is it?

The period 35—55 years — middle age — is a stage of transition. From full and vigorous, active youth the passage to ageing maturity includes the pre-maturity of middle age.

It is an important period of life because it is at this time that individual and personal actions can be taken to lay the foundations of a healthy old age. It is at this time that good habits can be laid and made for the future and bad habits given up.

It is a time of social, family, occupational, and personal change, as well as health and medical change.

It is a time when blissful, automatic, youthful acceptance of good health and well-nigh immortality is replaced by a realization that more than half the allotted span of three score and ten years has passed and that the downward slope with increasing physical restrictions and proneness to less than full health is being reached.

Normal changes

Certain changes are normal and inevitable at middle age. They have to be accepted gracefully and not resisted.

Physical changes

The most obvious change in women is the *menopause*, at which the ability to have children ceases. Simply, this is the result of all the unfertilized ova (eggs) in the ovaries having been used up. Accompanying this change is the cessation of monthly menstrual bleeding. Each monthly menses is the passage of ova from the ovaries down the uterine tubes into the uterus. If pregnancy does not take place then the unfertilized ovum is expelled with some of the uterine lining. The menopause is a normal and natural stage and need not and should not be associated with any dramatic physical, mental, or sexual changes. There is a range of recognized normal symptoms such as hot flushes and sweats, changed texture of skin and hair, tendency to muscular flabbiness and weight increase, and dryness of the vagina, but these tend to be compensated with time and with attention to food intake and maintenance of body exercise.

In *general* at this time physical capacity becomes less and one is less able to do things as quickly or as forcefully as in the past. This realization comes slowly but its implications must be heeded. The middle-aged labourer and sportsman discovers tricks in technique that enable him to achieve his objectives as well as, if less quickly than, his younger colleagues.

At this *pre-ageing* period there occur physical changes in the whole body. Eyesight and hearing become less acute, joints less flexible (unless actively maintained and exercised), weight increases (unless controlled), hair starts to thin, blood pressure creeps up, and memory becomes less nimble.

Mental changes

With middle age comes the acceptance of one's place in the world in general and in one's little world in particular. Revolutionary zeals and endeavours wane and there is less desire to change the world. Ambitions and expectations become more realistic and related to the possible rather than the unattainable impossible.

Women and to a lesser extent men, are prone to stress, tension, anxieties, and depression.

Social changes

Within the *family*, children are growing up and passing through adolescence and after, with all that it entails. They are leaving school, going on to further education, or starting work. They are having 'affairs'. They are becoming rebellious, recalcitrant, and self-reliant — but still in need of help, support, and some protection.

Parents, if they are still alive, are in their 70s and 80s and are beginning to cause problems. They become less able to live alone and need help. They may live some distance away. They may suffer acute medical or social crises.

Links with one's own *extended family* — brothers, sisters, cousins, in-laws, and others — tend to become tenuous and stretched and family gatherings become less common.

Work issues may create problems. Promotion and success take up much time for husband and wife. If both follow successful careers their problems may increase. Non-success is a source of depression and anxiety.

Housebound mothers become despondent at the frustration of continuing and never-ending housework.

Financial problems may ease if income increases, but there are family and other expenses that cause problems and with current inflation these problems grow.

Marital stresses may appear as a result of the external and internal changes, and breakdown and divorce are not uncommon results in middle age.

Leisure and social activities change from overactive to less active pursuits. Circles of friends become smaller and more intimate.

Habits become fixed and established and some are not good habits. Too much eating, too much drinking, too much smoking, and too little exercise are potential dangers for the future. This is the time to pause, think and correct such habits.

Common diseases

Middle age is a cross-roads of disease. Some problems and diseases are particularly prevalent in middle age, such as:

Backache.
Migraine.
Stomach and duodenal ulcers.
Anxiety and depression.
Urinary infections and gynaecological problems in women.

There are the beginnings of disorders of ageing and degeneration. These may affect some in middle age, such as:

High blood pressure.
Heart disease.
Strokes.
Cancers.
Bronchitis.
Rheumatism.
Chronic brain failure.

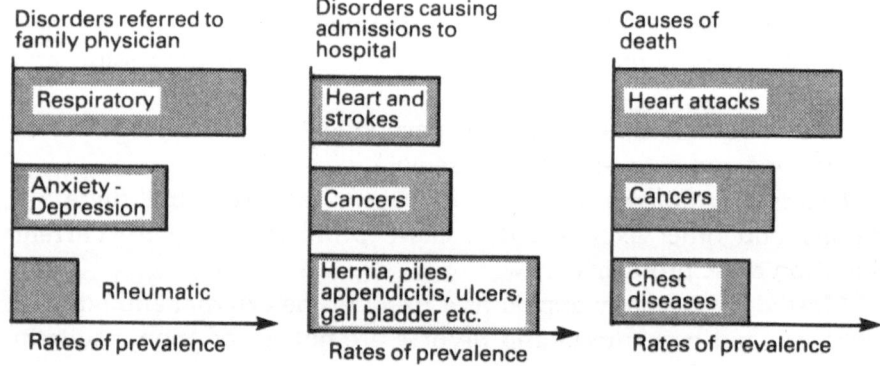

Figure 8.1 Common disorders of middle age.

For a diagrammatic insight to the common disorders of middle age Figure 8.1 shows those that commonly cause persons to consult their family physician, cause admission to hospital, and cause death.

From Figure 8.1 it is evident that disorders of the respiratory system such as coughs, colds, flu, bronchitis, and asthma are the most common reasons *for consulting the family physician*, followed by anxiety and depression, and then rheumatic problems such as backache, fibrositis, neuralgia, and arthritis.

Top reasons for *admission to hospitals* are conditions of the gastro-intestinal system — such as hernia, piles, ulcers, colitis, and gall bladder disorders — and cancers, followed in incidence by cancers and heart troubles.

Top *causes of death* in middle age are heart attacks from coronary artery disease, cancers, and bronchitis, emphysema, and pneumonia.

What risks and what to do about them?

At the cross-roads of middle age each one of us has to come face to face with realities. He or she has safely come through childhood, youth, and young adult life. Middle age is a time to take note of the present and prepare for the future.

Much of the future lies beyond our personal control. Some of it is influenced by our stock from previous generations. Some disorders are predestined and precast, such as high concentrations of blood fat that can cause extra risks to blockage of coronary arteries; diabetes; high blood pressure; strokes; and arthritis may be genetically influenced, as may some cancers. We cannot select our ancestors but we can help ourselves.

Many health risks relate to personal habits and personal environment and are correctable.

High among the potential risks on which we can take preventive actions are:

Excessive smoking of cigarettes.
Excessive eating and overweight.
Excessive consumption of alcohol.
Excessive indolence and lack of regular, energetic exercise.
Excessive stress and tension.
Excessive risks on the road, at work, and in the home.

What can be done?

There are a number of ways in which we can be more responsible for our own better health.

Better habits
As noted already, these are in our own hands. Outsiders, family, lay or professional, cannot live our lives for us. It is up to each of us to know what habits are potentially harmful and to avoid them.

Early symptoms of serious diseases
There are certain symptoms that may be of significance as early warnings of underlying disorders that are better treated early. It is up to the individual to learn to take note of these and then to collaborate

with his or her personal physician. Again it is our own responsibility, first, to take note and act, and, second, to collaborate.

Symptoms to be taken seriously are:

Bleeding from rectum, vagina, bladder, or coughing blood.
Unaccustomed breathlessness.
Persistent or recurrent pains in chest, abdomen, head, or anywhere else.
Unexpected loss or gain in weight.
Excessive tiredness.
Excessive thirst.
Any other that may cause anxiety.

Screening or medical check-up

These have a relatively little useful part to play in promoting better health. They may pick up abnormal readings in testing the blood, from X-rays or other tests, but the person usually has already noted symptoms.

It is wrong to expect such tests to correct problems or disorders that are in our own hands.

9

Pre- and post-retirement

What is 'retirement'?

One of the major turnings in life takes place at 'retirement'. But what is 'retirement'? It really is a euphemism for the transition from middle age to old age.

Retirement is a convenient social expedient for removing from work employed workers who reach certain ages. Note that mothers, grandmothers, housewives, and the self-employed do not 'retire'; they continue working.

There are so many invidious anomalies of retirement that it is obviously an illogical and farcical manoeuvre designed to benefit the younger workers by creating a promotion vacuum so that they can be sucked up into higher wage brackets.

Little account seems to be taken of the capabilities, abilities, or the wishes of those retiring. An age barrier is set and all who pass it are 'retired'.

Another anomaly is the different retiring age for men (usually 65) and women (usually at 60). For two reasons this is out of step with reality. First, women are by no means the weaker sex. They live longer than men; their life expectancy is 5–6 years above that of men. Second, with current moves towards sex equality, why this particular inequality? Apart from such social confusions and illogicalities, 'retirement' is a useful point for discussing old age and preparation for its arrival.

Old age

Everywhere in the world people are living longer. In Roman and
Norman times life expectancy was less than 40 years. Now, the likely
life expectancy of babies born in the 1980s should be well beyond the
biblical three-score-and-ten years. In countries such as Sweden, the
UK, and the USA, women can expect to live to 76—77 years and men to
72—73 years.

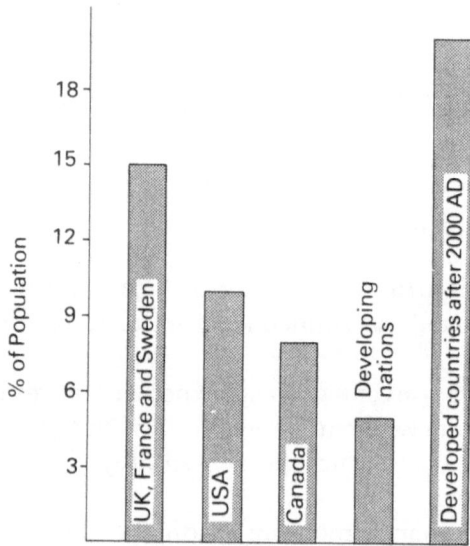

Figure 9.1   Proportions of population aged 65 or over.

With longer life, smaller families, and declining birth rates, the
proportions of elderly persons in our communities are increasing. In
Sweden, the UK, and France, the proportions of those aged 65 years
and over are over 15%; in the USA the proportion is 10%; in Canada it
is 8%; and in a developing country in Africa, Asia, or South America
it is below 5% (Figure 9.1). The proportion in developed countries is
likely to reach 20% by the year 2000. That means that one in five will
be retired and dependent on the rest of the population. It means, also,
that four out of five young adults can look forward to retiring and
experiencing the joys and problems of old age.

Amongst the elderly there are many more women than men and the difference becomes greater at higher ages. From a preponderance of women of 3 : 2 at 65 years the ratio reaches 2 : 1 at 85 and over. Old women outlive and outnumber men.

What is 'old age'?

There is no fair and acceptable definition of 'old age'. It has no set times and it is prone to considerable individual variations and expectations. No two persons age at the same rates and each person has his or her own attitude to, and expectations from, old age. Yet the body's changes with age are similar in most of us.

Ageing is a process of change shared by all of us, but within this common process there is a mixture of normal and abnormal changes. Some of the changes of ageing are inevitable, such as greying hair, wrinkling skin, and less-acute senses. Other changes may be the results of diseases that become increasingly likely with ageing such as rheumatism, heart and circulatory disorders, and strokes.

It is the combination between *physiology* (the normal processes of ageing) and *pathology* (the abnormal processes of disease) that create the patterns and pictures of old age. These combinations tend to have certain common and familiar presentations but there may be highly individual variations.

The *effects of ageing* can be put together under four sets of problems:

Effects on physical bodily functions.
Effects on mental and nervous behaviour.
Effects on social matters.
Effects leading to medical problems.

Changes — normal and abnormal

Retirement

Taking retirement as a normal but highly artificial moment of time there are certain inevitable changes that take place suddenly and dramatically.

From an independent, productive worker earning a regular income the retired person becomes a more dependent being relying on pension, savings, and any other income that he, or she, can acquire.

From being a self-confident breadwinner with little time to spare, retirement may lead to feelings of being a second-class citizen with much, often too much, time to fill.

If we are to go on living beyond our 70s and into our 80s, then as much as one fifth of our lives may be spent as 'retired', a period longer than our childhood.

Pre-retirement is an important period allowing time to think about, and prepare for, retirement. It is wise that our retirement plans and needs should be considered. Attention should be given to:

Health maintenance and disease avoidance by following basic rules of health.

Medical services — maintaining links with physicians and other local health services that one has developed.

Housing and living facilities — not moving to a retirement area dominated by old people unless one is confident that it will lead to more comfort, security, and happiness. Do not sever established roots with friends, family, and local services.

Leisure and social activities should be created; promoted, and developed to fill the time available during retirement.

Retirement should be looked on as the end of the beginning rather than as the beginning of the end.

Functional physical changes

Although the rates of ageing and the effects produced may be highly personal and variable certain changes are inevitable and have to be accepted and lived with.

As examples:

Physical ability declines — we cannot do at 65 what we could do at 45 or 55.

Work rates changes — crude physical work rate is lower but with age, effective and efficient short cuts can be developed and many highly delicate skills maintained.

Senses become less acute — vision alters and hearing is dulled, memory is less good and sharp.

Joints become less mobile, creaky, and painful at times.

Loss of height is usual due to some softening and shrinking of the spinal bones.

Weight may increase or fall.

Skin becomes less elastic and more wrinkled; bruising is more likely, especially on the arms and hands.

Hair becomes thinner, softer, and greyer.

Breathing may be more difficult on effort.

Digestive processes become less able to deal with certain foods and drinks.

There is less ability to deal with low and high external temperatures, i.e. with cold and hot weather.

Sleep patterns change with less sleep at night and more sleep in day.

Despite all these normal changes it is wrong to assume that most old persons are dull, disabled, and incapable. The following table shows just how few are bedfast and housefast, and how many are functionally able to carry on an independent existence.

Table 9.1   Percentages of those able, near-housebound, or disabled at three ages.

Age (years)	Able and independent	Near-housebound and in need of assistance	Disabled and bed- or chairbound
65	80	18	2
75	60	35	5
85	45	45	10

Mental changes

Ageing affects the brain as well as the body and certain changes occur gradually and imperceptibly.

Memory for recent events becomes poor but long-term memory remains good.

Forgetfulness and imprecision in daily affairs become noticeable.

Confusion may occur at times.

General mental slowing up.

Emotional instability and unusual liability to depression, anger, and bad temper.

Social changes

These are part of physical and other changes.

Society is more orientated to the speed and flair of youth and materialism, and the elderly have to strive for a place within a self-centred, selfish society.

With dependence on others some restrictions arise and increase unless prepared for and corrected.

Smaller families with wider geographical dispersal can lead to isolation and vulnerability.

Social mobility has increased and newly built estates are not conducive to deep-rooted neighbourliness.

Medical changes

These are related to the increased likelihood of suffering from conditions of ageing and degeneration, such as:

Diseases of heart and circulation, causing *heart failure and disorders of circulation of legs.*

Circulatory disease of the arteries of the brain, possibly leading to *strokes.*

The risk of *cancer* in some organs increases with age.

Joints tend to wear out with time, causing forms of *arthritis and rheumatism.*

Subjects with *chronic bronchitis and emphysema* tend to suffer more as they age.

Common problems and diseases

Certain basic medical facts are important in understanding good care for the elderly.

Whilst there is much that can be done to relieve many symptoms and whilst it is possible to cure some conditions it must be realized that 'cure' is not possible in most disorders affecting the elderly, since many of these are the results of processes of wear, tear, and degeneration.

Doctors tend to be trained in a 'single-pathology' approach. That is, they are encouraged to think in terms of a single disease causing the symptoms and problems and in terms of forms of treatment designed to treat that single cause. The elderly, however, can have a multiplicity of disorders at the same time and a *multiple-pathology* approach is necessary. An old person may have arthritis, heart failure, anaemia, diabetes, bronchitis, gastric ulcer, and depression all at the same time, and all may need diagnosis, assessment, and treatment.

Problems in the elderly may be the accumulated results of *long-standing diseases to which are added the burdens and stresses of a new disease* — thus an old lady may have suffered a stroke some years past and discovers a lump in her breast that turns out to be a tumour requiring treatment.

Old persons have *different responses and reactions* than younger people to pain, being less demonstrative and less complaining; to changes in temperature, their internal temperature-regulating mechanisms being less efficient so that they can suffer serious results from hypothermia (cold) or from heat stroke (hot); and they tend to react differently to common infections with less fever and fewer signs of local bodily reactions.

The *aims of treatment* in the elderly have somewhat different priorities than those in younger persons. Whilst attempts to *cure* should be made whenever possible this may not be feasible and efforts should be made to:

Maintain and restore the active *function and independence* of the elderly person.
Provide *relief* of unpleasant symptoms.
Provide human *care* and *comfort*.

Enthusiasm to cure and relieve by means of powerful modern drugs, surgery, or other hospital procedures must be tempered with the fact that such enthusiastic endeavours may lead to *complications and unpleasant effects of the treatment and investigations.*

Particular problems may result in the elderly from medical use of sleeping pills; of drugs for high blood pressure; of diuretics (drugs to increase output of urine), of sedatives, tranquillizers, and anti-depressants; of drugs for heart failure (such as digoxin and beta-blockers); of the many drugs for rheumatism and arthritis; and of drugs for Parkinson's disease.

Senility

This is an unhelpful and unfair label. It tends to be applied to old persons with *brain failure* — that is, those whose mental state has become disturbed. Memory may have become poor, there is confusion and disorientation, restlessness, unusual behaviour, wandering out alone, lack of cleanliness, dirty habits, and general inability to cope and care for themselves.

This state of *dementia* (brain failure) may be the result of circulatory changes affecting the brain (mini-strokes) or from other internal diseases such as cancers, diabetes or others, from ill effects of prescribed medicines, from over-indulgence in alcohol, or from a state of primary depression.

Specific diseases

It is not possible to go into great detail of the many diseases which may afflict the elderly but some need to be mentioned.

Rheumatism may be the result of worn and arthritic joints (some, such as hip joints, can now be replaced with artificial prostheses with great benefits), but painful limbs, backaches, and neckaches may be caused by: gout, polymyalgia (an inflammation of muscles that responds dramatically to cortisone-type preparations); and internal diseases such as thyroid deficiency, cancers, or bone diseases.

Heart failure may lead to breathlessness, black-outs, or swollen legs — but not all swollen legs are due to serious heart or kidney disorders, and not all 'funny turns' are related to serious heart disorders.

Breathlessness may be the consequence of heart diseases such as blocked coronary arteries or high blood pressure, but also it may result from bronchitis and asthma or even from anaemia due to malnourishment.

Incontinence of urine and/or faeces is a degrading and serious problem for all who have to care for the elderly. Usually associated with brain failure and immobility, from confinement to bed, it can at times be associated with disease within the bladder or rectum or from such an easily correctable condition as faecal impaction (constipation with accumulation of excessive amounts of hard faeces in the rectum which the old person cannot expel alone and which need removing by a nurse).

Care of the dying: 'The mortality of life is 100 per cent'. We shall all die. Some will die quickly and without suffering, yet others may linger long and require much care.

Care of the dying depends in detail on the causal disease but more generally they need:

Emotional and spiritual support and loving care.

Relief from physical discomfort by good nursing and medication.

Support of the family and friends during bereavement, with sensitive understanding.

Principles of care of the elderly

There are no secret universally successful ways of caring for the elderly.

The elderly must be encouraged to live as full and as independent an existence as possible.

As back-up there should be regular contacts with family, friends, neighbours, or community services to ensure that extra care and support can be available when required.

Depending on functional state the elderly person may live in their own homes, sheltered accommodation with warden or other support, nursing homes, or hospital.

Wherever they live there is need for an organization of community medical and social services that can be called upon for extra help when required. These may be:

Medical care from family physician, nurses, and hospital.

Help in the home from home-help, meals-on-wheels, and structural aids in the home.

Clubs and day centres for social, meal, and other activities.

Housing facilities appropriate to needs.

Money and other material assistance.

10
Health resources and how to use them

Common diseases

There is a gradation of severity among common diseases. Fortunately, most of our non-health problems and diseases are minor and self-limiting, with few risks of permanent damage.

It is estimated that of all non-health problems in the community at any time:

65% are *minor and self-limiting.*

25% are concerned with *chronic disorders* such as rheumatism, chest troubles, depression, heart and circulatory troubles, and others.

10% are caused by *serious major and life-threatening diseases*, such as cancer, strokes, effects of heart attacks, pneumonia, and others.

Levels of care

Accepting as facts this gradation of disease all health care systems have four clearly recognizable levels of care (Figure 10.1). These levels are essential and inevitable and are found in every national health system be it in the USA, the USSR, the UK, Spain, China, India, Africa, Australia or developing countries. These four levels are:

147

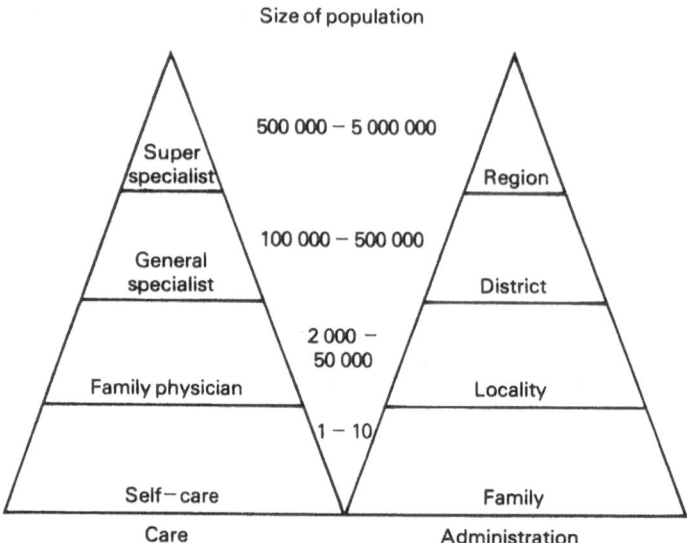

Figure 10.1   Levels of medical care.

Self-care — care by the individual and family for minor and trivial ailments by home remedies or through self-medication with drugs obtained at a pharmacy.

Primary professional care — which may be from medical or non-medical sources. Medical primary care may be given by family physicians, general practitioners or other physicians. Alternatively, it may be provided by nurses or social workers.

General specialist care — tends to be based on a district with centralized general hospital resources. The specialists that are available provide treatment for internal medical, general surgical, paediatric, obstetric—gynaecological, accident and orthopaedic, and psychiatric problems. In addition there have to be facilities for radiological and pathological investigations. Other specialties may be available on a visiting basis, such as for eyes, ear, nose, and throat; skin, rheumatology and others.

Super-specialist care — medical specialization has advanced so fast and so far that there are increasing numbers of super-specialists that care for the more rare and more complex medical problems, such as

treatment for leukaemia and other rare cancers (oncology), neuro-
surgery, heart surgery, plastic surgery, and others. Such units need to
be few and each based to serve large populations (1—5 million).

Flow of care

Although the structures of a national health care system vary and
depend on national politics, wealth and economics, philosophies,
culture and geography, the flow of care is similar, with some local
characteristics (Figure 10.2).

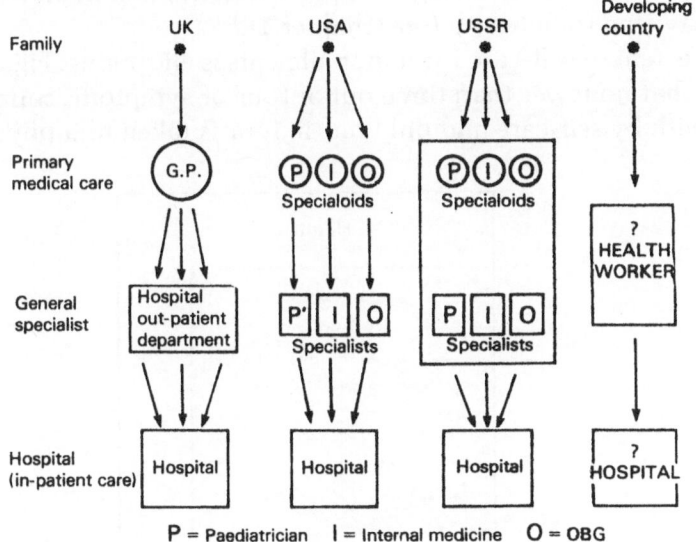

Figure 10.2 Flow of medical care.

The *British NHS* is based historically on primary care being
provided by general practitioners and it is their general practitioner to
whom the people go in the first instance. It is the general practitioner
who refers patients to specialists and hospital services.

The *US system* is much less organized and there never has been a
strong concept of a single family physician caring for the whole family.
The American can, and does, go to a variety of physicians for primary
care.

In the *USSR* the system is rigidly organized and is based on poly-
clinics that provide both primary and general specialist facilities.

Self-care

Self-care is essential in all systems of health care. No system could provide completely professional care for every ache, sneeze, or ill feeling.

It is only right that the public should provide a considerable amount of self-care and to accept considerable responsibilities for maintaining health and preventing disease. For there is much more to self-care than self-medication.

Health maintenance requires an understanding of the nature of health promotion, following the rules of health, and avoiding habits that may lead to ill health (see Chapter 1).

The extent of self-care for minor ailments is enormous. Figure 10.3 shows that no fewer than three out of four of symptoms suffered are dealt with by self-care and only one in four is taken to a physician.

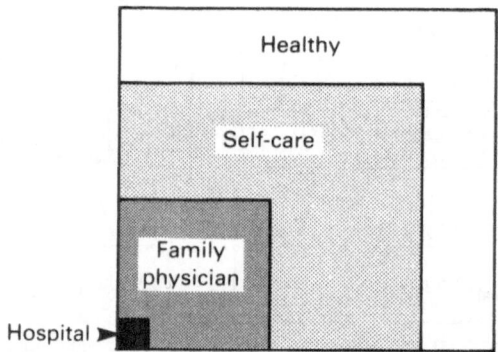

Figure 10.3   Proportion of population in good health, administering self-care, receiving care from general physician, or receiving care in hospital.

Much of self-care for minor illness is through self-medication. At any time in the USA, UK and Europe, and Australasia, almost two thirds of all persons are taking some medication. Of this huge amount of medication one half — one in three of the population — is taking prescribed medicines and one in three consuming non-prescribed medicines obtained over the counter from a pharmacy.

The five most popular OTC (over-the-counter) medicines purchased by the public are:

Analgesics (aspirin, paracetamol, and similar products).
Vitamins (as tonics).
Cough medicines.
Skin applications.
Laxatives.

Self-care and self-medication are important but neglected subjects. Both should be better understood by the public. Both should be taught in schools and through continuing public education and information in the public media.

Primary professional care

When the need to seek professional medical advice arises one must know who to consult, how to do so, where, and when.

Primary professional medical care is based on a locality and it must be one of the regular neighbourhood services. It is as essential as the local food store and should be within reasonable, easy access.

Good primary care is the basis for good health care as a whole. It is useless having good, expensive hospitals if primary health care is poor, flimsy, and unreliable.

The content and the process of primary care are similar everywhere but detailed organization varies. Thus in the UK all persons are entitled to, and are, registered under the National Health Service (NHS), with a general practitioner of their choice. It is to that general practitioner that they go when they need any medical advice. It is not possible in the UK under the NHS to go direct to a specialist. It is the custom for a person requiring specialist care to be referred by their general practitioner.

The general practitioner in the UK and his colleagues in other countries provides:

An available and accessible 24-hour service — if he or she is off duty another member of the team will provide cover.

First-contact care where the patient's problems are assessed and managed.

Co-ordination of local medical and social services. It is the general practitioner who knows what is available locally and which services should be brought into action. These services include nursing, welfare, social, home help, and other services.

Long-term and continuing care. It is through such long-term relationships that patients and physician come to know and to respect each other.

The principles of primary care are similar in other countries. In the USA the family select their own coterie of primary physicians who are specialists as internists, obstetricians/gynaecologists, paediatricians, and psychiatrists.

In the USSR there is a limited choice of services and physicians. There is a primary care team allocated to each locality and it is to the team in the local polyclinic that the person goes when in need of care.

General specialist care

The most likely conditions for which hospitalization is required are:

Surgical operations for hernia, varicose veins, appendicitis, breast lumps, skin cysts, and haemorrhoids.

Medical problems such as heart attacks, drug overdose, pneumonia and bronchitis, strokes, high blood pressure, and investigation of dyspepsia and other conditions.

Paediatric problems of development, and of infections.

Traumatic, orthopaedic, and rheumatic disorders.

Psychiatric disorders such as depression, anxiety, stress, and problems of the elderly.

Maternity services and management of *gynaecological disorders.*

Patients with these conditions are referred to the general specialists by primary physicians; the general district hospital service has the necessary facilities and resources.

Super-specialist care

Increasing specialization demands a regional organization of super-specialist units to care for some conditions, such as:

Kidney diseases that may require dialysis or transplantation.

Brain and nervous disorders that may need very special investigation and treatment.

Chest and heart disorders that need very special assessment and possibly open-chest and heart surgery.

Others, such as eye disorders; ear, nose, and throat; deformities and disfigurements; joint diseases.

It is most economical and most efficient to centralize such expensive and complex services in regional or national units serving large populations.

How to use resources

To find one's way through the hazardous medical jungle an experienced guide is necessary. The best guide should be a well-known and respected family physician who knows the problems, the specialist services available, and who is best able to match the specialist to the needs of the patient.

PART II

11

Rheumatic diseases

Rheumatism is one of the most used of medical words. However, 'rheumatism' is a vague umbrella term; to some it represents any vague ache or pain, to others it conjures up a vision of a crippled invalid in a wheelchair.

Part of the problem is that the rheumatic disorders affect the connective tissues which are found in every part of the body. These tissues form muscles, tendons, ligaments, joints and bones — all concerned with movements and activities. These structures can be strained, sprained, broken or fractured, dislocated or otherwise damaged by trauma. Joints may become mechanically deranged, they may degenerate with age, or they may become inflamed or infected. Any or all of these processes occurring anywhere in the body may give rise to 'rheumatism'.

Their importance does not lie in any threat to life, as a cause of death they are exceedingly rare. Rather it is the large amount of pain and suffering, disability, and loss of time from work which makes them important. In addition, the lack of really effective treatment in many of these disorders and the often spontaneous tendency to improvement with time leaves the field wide open for the exploitation of patients by those who are interested in making large amounts of money out of their suffering and gullibility.

Rheumatic disorders tend to become more common with increasing age (Figure 11.1).

157

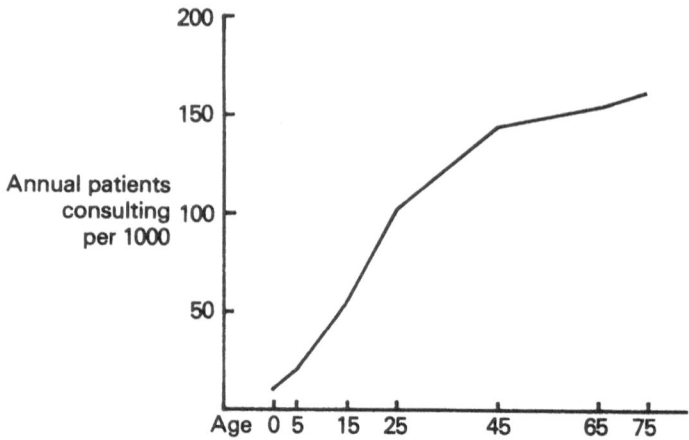

Figure 11.1   Incidence of rheumatic disorders with age.

Many minor rheumatic conditions are ignored or self-treated. Of those which are brought to a physician, the most common area of complaint is *backache* and the most likely causes of this are mechanical derangement and degeneration of the spine. The neck and shoulders are similarly but rather less often affected. Next in importance is *osteoarthritis* of the larger joints, especially the hips and knees. This is a degenerative process aggravated by wear and tear on the joint surfaces. Inflammatory conditions, where there is an active disease process occurring within the joints, occurs in less common disorders such as gout and rheumatoid arthritis; they account for less than 10% of all the rheumatic conditions seen by the physician.

Spinal problems — necks and backs

The *spine* consists of a column of rectangular bones which supports the skull at the top, the rib cage in the middle, and joins the pelvis at its lower end. It protects and encloses the spinal cord which extends down from the brain. Nerves pass out from the spinal cord between each pair of vertebrae to every part of the body. Each vertebra articulates with the vertebrae above and below. The whole structure is held together by ligaments and muscles in a complex network. Between adjacent vertebrae a pad of cartilage or gristle acts as a shock absorber. This is the notorious 'disc' which is alleged to 'slip' from time to time.

Since any of the various structures mentioned above may be damaged it is perhaps not surprising that the precise nature and location of the damage occurring when someone complains of pain in the neck and back is often difficult to determine accurately. Although X-rays can sometimes be helpful they show only the bones, and are most useful in excluding more serious conditions such as infections or cancer in the bones.

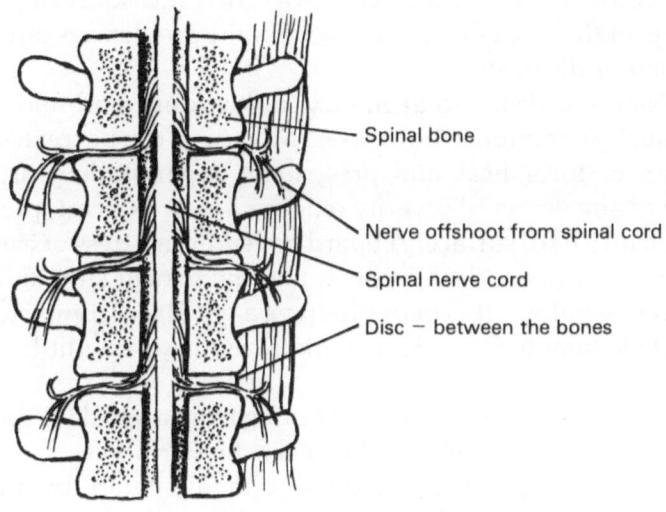

Spinal bone

Nerve offshoot from spinal cord

Spinal nerve cord

Disc — between the bones

Figure 11.2   Structure of the spine.

Problems in the neck are usually of two types. Young people may wake up with an *acute wryneck* which is painful to move. This may be helped by manipulation in the early stages but will settle on its own within a few days. Older people suffer recurrent attacks of neck pain from *cervical spondylosis*, a degenerative condition with roughening of the edges of the neck vertebrae, which leads to pressure on the nerve roots as they emerge from the spine. Sometimes this may cause pain and tingling down into the hands and arms. These attacks can be relieved by rest and pain-relieving drugs, often with the addition of a supporting collar and sometimes by traction, i.e. stretching of the neck, or other forms of physiotherapy.

Pain in the lower back, *lumbago*, is even more common. Typically, the victim is seized with a sudden pain in the lower back whilst lifting a heavy object, or the pain arises more gradually after unaccustomed exercise such as gardening. However, many people develop backache without any obvious precipitating cause. The backache may be associated with pain radiating into the buttock, thigh, and down as far as the foot. This is the area served by the sciatic nerve and the condition is known as *sciatica*. This suggests that the nerve root has been trapped by a piece of the intervertebral disc which has been squeezed out from between two lumbar vertebrae. It is this squeezing out, or prolapsing, of the disc which is the cause of the problem. A disc cannot actually slip or dislocate.

Acute back problems occur mostly in the young and middle aged and are equally common in both sexes. Mild cases can be treated by the application of local heat and prescribing a pain-killing drug, but back pain of any degree of severity requires a period of rest, preferably lying down on a hard surface. A board under the mattress or a mattress on the floor makes an ideal support, and the patient should have no more than one pillow. It is better to have a few days' complete rest at an early stage than to struggle on with increasing pain until forced to stop.

In most cases a period of strict rest lasting from a few days up to 3—4 weeks in a severe case will help the backache to resolve.

Some acute back problems respond to manipulation by an osteopath, physiotherapist, or doctor skilled in the technique, and longer standing problems may be helped by traction, physiotherapy, or wearing a corset, together with advice about obesity, lifting, and general back care. Very rarely an operation may be required for intractable pain from a severely damaged disc. Remember that, in nearly all cases of backache, the application of the measures outlined above will lead to a resolution of the problem within a few weeks at most.

Osteoarthritis

This is predominantly a condition of ageing of vulnerable joints. 95% of people over 65 have evidence of the condition on radiography but, luckily, many will have little or no symptoms and will require no treatment. It is twice as common in women as in men.

The joints most affected are those most exposed to the wear and tear of everyday use and also those which have been previously damaged by trauma or another disease process. Thus hands and feet and knees and hips are vulnerable, especially in persons who are overweight. The spinal joints may also become osteoarthritic, as may the shoulders, elbows, and wrists.

The affected joints become stiff, swollen, and painful and movements of the joints are restricted. Pain may be relieved by pain-killing drugs and in some cases physiotherapy and the use of a stick or walking-aid may help. Considerable progress has been made in surgically replacing damaged joints, especially the hips. However, the procedure is a major one and the patient needs to be in good health generally if he or she is to be able to withstand the operation and subsequent intensive physiotherapy.

Gout

Uric acid is a product of the body's metabolism. Some have difficulty in removing it from their bodies, so the blood contains too much uric acid. In certain circumstances uric acid crystals form in the joints giving rise to sudden, severe pain in the affected joint. It tends to occur first after the age of 40, much more often in men than women, and there is often a familial tendency. It is one of the very few rheumatic conditions for which we have an effective, specific treatment and where the patient may be confidently assured that the condition can be controlled and the attack of pain abolished.

It is most important that the patient understands the condition and complies with the treatment responsibly since the drug, allopurinol, which enables the body to excrete the uric acid and prevent further attacks, can itself precipitate acute gout in the early stages of treatment. The acute attack is controlled by an anti-inflammatory drug such as indomethacin.

Rheumatoid arthritis

Rheumatoid arthritis is a generalized disorder which can affect the whole body, often making the patient feel generally unwell and tired. It is thought to be caused by a disturbance of the body's own immunity system, in which normal body tissues are mistakenly identified as foreign protein and attacked and damaged. This process is vital in protecting us against bacteria and viruses, but causes problems when organs such as kidneys or heart are transplanted. The phenomenon of the body attacking its own tissues is known as autoimmunity.

Although it is a generalized disease it is the damage to the joints which is the characteristic feature of rheumatoid arthritis. It may occur at any age but it is most common in the 35—55 year age group and is three times as common in women as in men. A family physician can expect to see two or three new cases yearly and is likely to be looking after 12—20 patients with the condition at any one time. Although it is a potentially serious condition, which can cause prolonged pain and serious disability, this is by no means an inevitable outcome. Over a period of years about one third of patients become severely disabled and crippled by this disease, whilst another third will have continuing problems and symptoms which interfere with normal functioning. The other 30—40%, however, will have little continuing pain or residual disability and the disease is said to have burnt itself out.

Rheumatoid arthritis generally has a slow, insidious onset with transient pain and stiffness in muscles and joints, particularly those of the hands, wrists, knees, and elbows. Characteristically, joints on both sides of the body are affected together. Stiffness and pain in the morning or after resting are likely, and tend to improve gradually with use. Perhaps one in five has a more dramatic onset and feels ill with loss of appetite and weight and a more sudden onset of joint pain. Blood tests and X-rays will help to confirm the diagnosis and plan appropriate treatment.

What to do

There is at present no known method of preventing rheumatoid arthritis. There is also no specific cure available, despite the regular announcements of new wonder drugs and dramatic breakthroughs. However, much can be done to relieve pain, improve mobility, and minimize disability. This requires close co-operation between the patient and his or her family, the physician and the specialist services provided by the hospital and the social services.

Initially, the family physician will confirm the diagnosis, prescribe the appropriate drugs to relieve pain and inflammation, and help the patient to understand the need for appropriate resting of the affected joints, combined with gentle exercises to prevent permanent stiffness. Many milder cases can be managed perfectly satisfactorily in this way, often with the help of the district nurse. In more serious cases arrangements may be made to consult a specialist. He or she may need to admit the patient to hospital for further tests or intensive physiotherapy. He or she may also prescribe more powerful drugs such as gold or penicillamine which have a specific action in reducing joint inflammation in rheumatoid arthritis. However, they require close monitoring with blood and urine tests since they may cause serious side effects.

In some patients injections of cortisone into the affected joints may be effective, and surgical removal of the affected joint linings may also help.

Ultimately, a seriously affected patient may need occupational therapy or require retraining for new employment. Structural alterations may be required to the home and various aids to daily living provided. The support and encouragement of the patient by his or her family is absolutely vital if a good outcome is to be obtained.

Other rheumatic disorders

Many of the rheumatic conditions seen by the family physician do not fit neatly into a specific diagnosis. Many chronic inflammations such as *tennis elbow*, *capulitis* of the shoulder, and *housemaid's knee* can be relieved by rest and pain relief, and sometimes by the injection of cortisone into the affected area.

An important condition affecting the elderly is *polymyalgia rheumatica* in which the muscles of the shoulder and hip regions become stiff and painful. In some of these cases the patients develop *cranial arteritis* which can threaten the eyesight and these conditions respond dramatically to cortisone.

Ankylosing spondylitis is becoming recognized as a much more common disorder than was previously suspected and it has been found to be associated with a particular tissue type, somewhat akin to blood grouping. In this condition, which predominantly affects young men, the most important part of treatment is active physiotherapy and exercise to prevent the spine stiffening to force the patient into a permanently bent, flexed position.

Conclusion

It is the physician's responsibility in all types of rheumatic disorders to sort out those which need specific investigation and treatment from those which will settle spontaneously. The patient can help enormously by co-operating intelligently with the treatment programme and making the best use of the considerable resources. There is no good evidence that special diets, the wearing of copper bracelets or red flannel, faith healing, or taking the waters at a famous spa have any beneficial effects. However, there is no reason to discourage these activities so long as they do no harm. Osteopathy is certainly helpful in some cases and acupuncture is at present under serious investigation in the West after some dramatic demonstrations by Chinese physicians.

It is unlikely that there will ever be a single, specific treatment for all rheumatic conditions. However, if that should ever come about it will preclude the vast range of methods of treatment offered at present. There were many choices of treatment for pneumonia before penicillin was discovered — now there is only one!

12

Gastrointestinal diseases

Disorders of the gastrointestinal (or digestive) system are an important and sizeable cause of illness. They account for about 10% of all consultations in family practice and for more than 10% of all hospital admissions and deaths. However, it is usually only the more troublesome or persistent symptoms that reach the physician as it is likely that

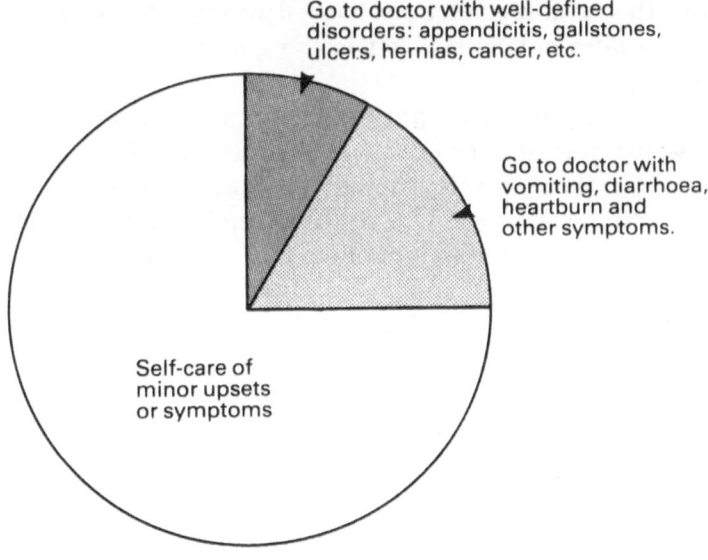

Figure 12.1 Consultation pattern for gastrointestinal disease.

165

everyone will experience some kind of minor digestive upset during the course of a year and be able to manage it themselves.

Of those who do consult the physician about two-thirds do so with minor conditions such as acute infections with sickness and diarrhoea or vague symptoms such as heartburn, indigestion, 'wind', constipation, and less than one-third with well-defined disorders such as piles, peptic ulcers, hernias, gallbladder disease, cancer, and acute appendicitis or other emergencies (see Figure 12.1)

Structure and function (see Figure 12.2)

Second only to the respiratory (breathing) system the gastrointestinal tract is in almost continual use. Foods and liquids in all their various forms enter the digestive system through the mouth and then undergo a series of complex processes designed to extract from them those parts which the body needs for its own growth and energy requirements. Carbohydrate (for energy), protein (for building tissues), fat (for energy and stores), minerals, and vitamins are all dealt with in different ways though in accordance with the same underlying principle. Namely, that which the body needs is broken down in the gut and then absorbed through its wall into the bloodstream, and what the body does not need is left in the gut to be ejected in the bowel motion.

Germs and potentially poisonous or cancer-producing substances are also ingested and the body has to protect itself against them. Acid produced in the stomach generally kills off the germs — if it does not then infection can result. Dietary fibre (indigestible vegetable matter) in the diet increases the weight of the faeces, dilutes the contents of the bowel, speeds up the time it takes for food to go through the bowel, and so lessens the possible contact between cancer-producing substances and the bowel wall. In underdeveloped countries where, unlike here, a lot of fibre-rich foods are eaten the incidence of cancer of the bowel and other major bowel diseases is less and it is thought that the high-fibre diet may be protective.

In the *mouth* chewing breaks up large food particles and mixes the food with saliva which moistens it and starts the digestive process. Swallowing takes the food down the oesophagus or gullet through a sphincter, or valve, into the stomach. This sphincter stops the stomach

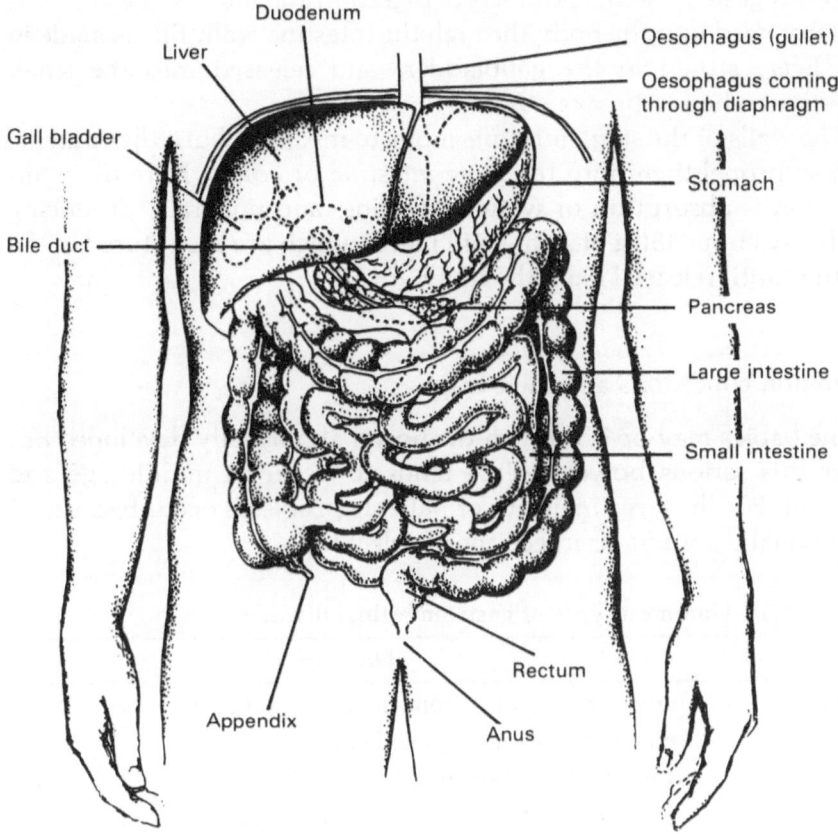

Figure 12.2 Structure of the gastrointestinal tract.

contents from coming back up and if it does not work properly then heartburn or indigestion can ensue.

Food is stored in the *stomach*, mixed with acid, mucus, and the digestive enzyme pepsin and then released at a controlled, steady rate into the duodenum where it is digested further and absorbed. Too much acid in some people may lead to duodenal ulcers while too little may lead to gastric ulcers.

The *duodenum* is the first part of a long tube called the small intestine. Here the partly digested food is mixed with bile, pancreatic secretions, and the secretions of the bowel wall itself to become completely digested. All the products of digestion and most of the vitamins are absorbed into the body through the intestine wall. Bile is made in the liver, stored in the gallbladder, and released into the small intestine, where it breaks down fat.

The walls of the *small intestine* move to mix and churn the contents and so propel them into the *large intestine* or *colon*. Here the main function is absorption of water, vitamins, and minerals, producing each day about 150 g of semi-solid faeces which are then stored in the rectum until released from the body.

Common conditions and their causes

Some babies may be born with the bowel abnormally developed but after this serious bowel disease tends to occur in middle age and beyond. For the large majority of patients problems occur because of functional disorders or infections (Table 12.1).

Table 12.1   Common types of gastrointestinal diseases

Age group	Diseases
Babies	Infections, hernias, congenital abnormalities.
1+	Infections, worms, appendicitis.
20+	A little bit of everything.
50+	Hernias, hiatus hernias, gallstones, diverticulitis, cancer of the bowel.

Loss of appetite

This can occur as part of any kind of illness. If temporary it is of little significance but if persisting and associated with weight loss then it needs looking into.

Nausea and vomiting

These can occur as part of many different illnesses, especially in children. They are more likely to be significant if associated with constipation than with diarrhoea.

Flatulence (burping)

The expulsion of air which has been sucked into the oesophagus. It may be deliberate or come from eating radishes or cucumbers, or drinking alcohol. It may be a sign of an ulcer, hiatus hernia, or gall-stones but in a large group of people it occurs because they swallow with their mouths open. These people are often anxious and if they keep sucking a pen cap they will stop burping.

Flatus (farting)

This is passed about ten times a day by normal individuals. Increased amounts come from diet factors, such as eating beans, carrots, or turnips.

Heartburn/indigestion

This may be a sign of disease of the oesophagus or stomach but is more likely to be the result of dietary indiscretion or tension. If developing for the first time when older, then this may need investigating.

Abdominal pain

If occurring acutely, this is more likely to have a serious than a trivial cause and in the absence of vomiting and diarrhoea may well need looking into.

Diarrhoea

A frequent consequence of a bowel infection or dietary indiscretion and should last only for a few days. If it persists, keeps recurring, or is associated with the passage of blood or slime then it may be from a more serious underlying cause and would warrant investigation.

Constipation

False self-diagnosis is too often made. Normal bowels may move once a day or once a week and in the absence of discomfort need nothing to help them move. A lifelong high-fibre diet will help relieve true constipation greatly. Chronic constipation does not signify bowel disease but a change in bowel habit with recent constipation, especially in middle age or beyond, may well be more serious.

Diseases

Gastroenteritis (vomiting and diarrhoea)

This is most common in infancy and childhood but can affect all ages. It occurs all the year round and occasionally in epidemics, which may be due to food poisoning. In most cases the exact cause cannot be pinpointed although it is presumed that bacteria and viruses are responsible.

There may be vomiting, diarrhoea (together or alone), griping tummy ache, and a fever with a general feeling of being unwell. Infection is generally short and sharp, lasting 48—72 hours. Dehydration (depletion of body fluids) is a danger, especially in infants, and may occur if they have frequent and profuse vomiting or diarrhoea or if symptoms are prolonged for more than 24 hours.

Most attacks need no special treatment. Solid food should be avoided for 1—2 days, with plentiful clear fluids taken followed by a gradual return to normal eating as symptoms settle and appetite returns. Mixtures or tablets to stop the diarrhoea may be counterproductive, as symptoms can be prolonged by them and return when the medicine is stopped. Similarly, antibiotics can prolong infection, apart from having no effect against viruses and from being able to produce vomiting and diarrhoea as a side effect, and so should be avoided.

Hiatus hernia

This may develop in middle age. The oesophageal sphincter ceases to function properly and stomach acid and contents are allowed to go up into the oesophagus. This causes severe heartburn, especially on stooping or lying down at night. The main abnormality is caused by the stomach herniating through the diaphragm into the chest (see Figure 12.3).

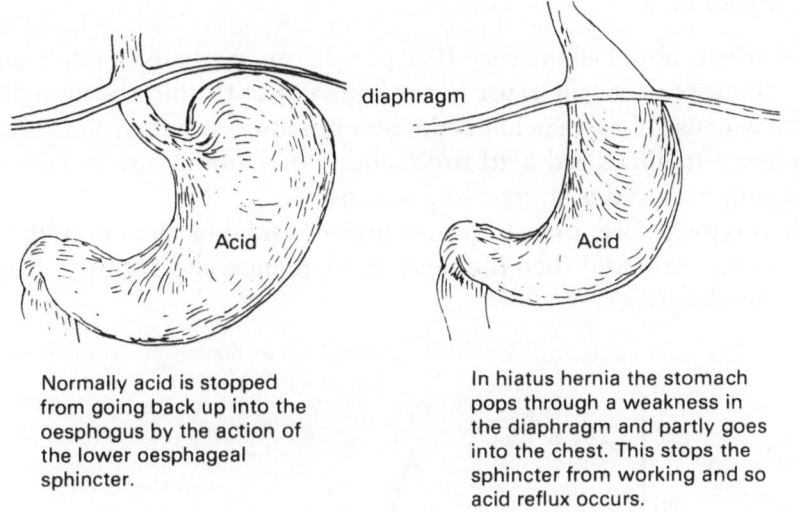

Normally acid is stopped from going back up into the oesphogus by the action of the lower oesphageal sphincter.

In hiatus hernia the stomach pops through a weakness in the diaphragm and partly goes into the chest. This stops the sphincter from working and so acid reflux occurs.

Figure 12.3 Hiatus hernia — mechanism.

Although inconvenient this is not a serious disorder and as symptoms may be persistent it is worthwhile following the simple measures for relief shown in Table 12.2.

Table 12.2 Measures to relieve heartburn, indigestion, and hiatus hernia

Stop smoking
Lose weight
Eat smaller meals
Eat less fatty foods
Avoid chocolate, coffee, alcohol, and acidic fruit drinks
Avoid tight garments, low chairs
Raise bed head 8—11 inches (20—28 cm)

Antacids (acid neutralizing mixtures or tablets, many varieties of which can be bought or prescribed) can be taken as often as necessary to help relieve symptoms. As a last resort in a few persistent and severe cases an operation to replace and tether the stomach fully in the abdomen may be performed.

Duodenal ulcer

This affects about 40 in every 1000 people, mainly between the ages of
20—40 years. The true cause is not known, but the ulcer is thought to
form because of extra acid production possibly coming from a family
tendency to increased acid production, or from excessive cigarette
smoking or nervous stresses and strains.

In a typical case, once begun, symptoms tend to recur periodically
for 5—10 years and then diminish in frequency and severity, finally
ceasing altogether.

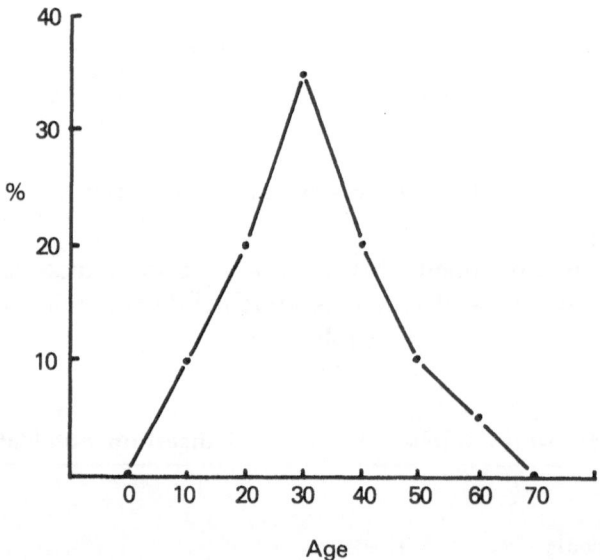

Figure 12.4   Duodenal ulcer — age at onset.

The *pain* is dull and gnawing in the pit of the stomach. It tends to
occur 1—2 hours after a meal and may wake the victim in the early
hours of the morning. It is relieved by eating, drinking milk, or taking
antacids. It does not usually affect the appetite or cause vomiting.
Attacks come in bouts for a few weeks and then may go away for a
variable length of time.

A *barium meal* may be necessary to confirm the diagnosis as may

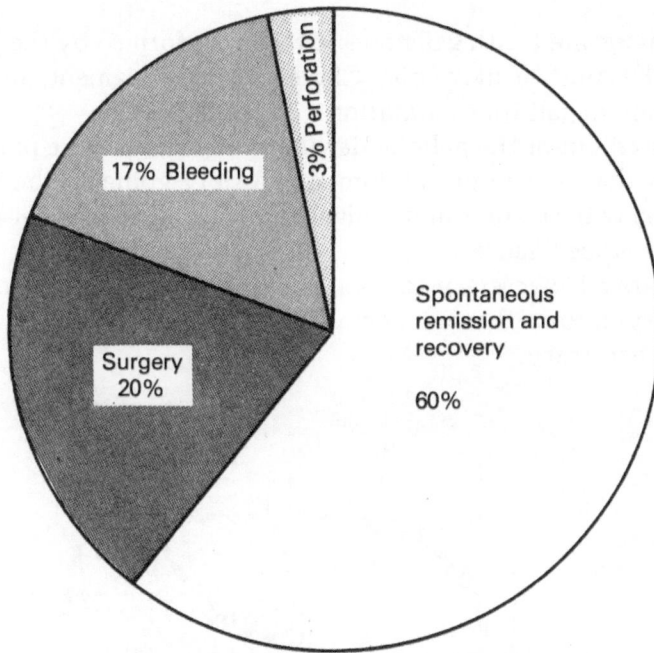

Figure 12.5 Duodenal ulcer — cause and outcome.

endoscopy (a fibre-optic instrument passed down the oesphagus to give a clear view of the inside of the stomach). The *main treatment* is medical and antacids taken liberally whenever necessary will control symptoms. They act quickly to relieve pain by chemically neutralizing the acid.

Avoiding smoking, alcohol, and aspirin-containing medicines may help but bed rest, regular time off work and strict diets do not appear to help. Small, frequent meals taken with plenty of milk may help as they have an acid-neutralizing effect.

If these measures are not successful a new drug called cimetidine (Tagamet) reduces the production of stomach acid and can be more effective. In those few cases where symptoms are severe and persistent (about 20%) and in those where complications of bleeding or perforation of the ulcer may occur (20%), surgery may be required to remove the ulcer or stop the stomach producing excessive acid.

Gallbladder disease

This is associated with gallstones. Stones are formed by the precipitation of the constituents of bile. Cholesterol, bile pigment, and calcium participate in gallstone formation.

If passed out of the gallbladder they can cause severe pain (biliary colic) in the right upper abdomen (possibly going to the back and shoulder) with sickness and indigestion. They may also get stuck and cause *jaundice* (Figure 12.6).

An X-ray is necessary for diagnosis and if gallstones are causing serious symptoms then an operation to remove the gallbladder may become necessary.

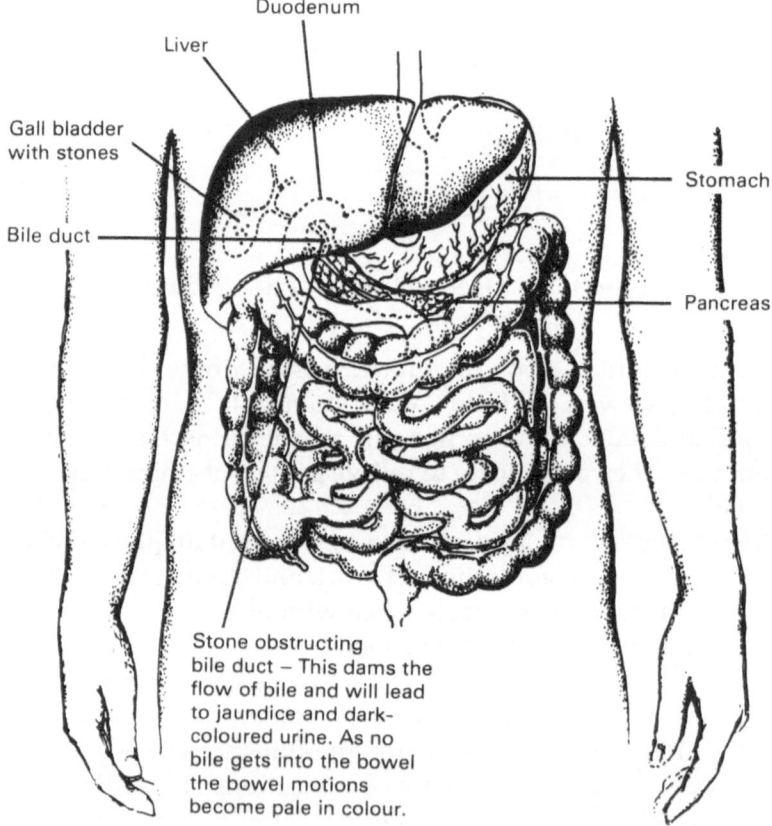

Duodenum

Liver

Gall bladder
with stones

Bile duct

Stomach

Pancreas

Stone obstructing
bile duct – This dams the
flow of bile and will lead
to jaundice and dark-
coloured urine. As no
bile gets into the bowel
the bowel motions
become pale in colour.

Figure 12.6   Biliary tract with gallstones.

Jaundice

This is caused by increased concentrations of bile pigment in the blood, producing yellowness of the whites of the eyes and skin, dark urine, and pale stools. In children and young adults it is usually caused by an infectious form of liver disease (infectious hepatitis), while in middle age and beyond it is more likely to be caused by gallstones or cancer of part of the pancreas. It may also occur as a side effect of some drugs if they damage the liver.

Appendicitis

This is inflammation of the appendix and may occur at any age, though it is most usual in children and young adults.

The history is usually fairly typical with nausea, loss of appetite, and vague central abdominal pain to begin with, followed by increasing severe and constant pain which settles in the right lower abdomen (see Figure 12.2 for the position of the appendix). At this stage a fever is usual and there may be some vomiting.

Once the diagnosis is suspected hospital admission for an operation is necessary, since the inflamed appendix may rupture internally and spill its infected contents causing peritonitis (inflammation of the lining of the abdomen).

Hernias

These are caused by weaknesses between muscles allowing the contents of the abdomen to protrude. They occur mainly at the umbilicus and in the groins. They can also occur internally, e.g. hiatus hernia is caused by the upper part of the stomach sliding through the diaphragm (a muscle) into the lower chest (see Figure 12.3 and page 68).

They are not dangerous unless they strangulate — i.e. unless bowel becomes nipped at the neck of the hernia, causing strangulation of the bowel tissues, perforation, and peritonitis. In this situation an urgent operation is required to release the strangulation and repair the hernia. In inguinal, femoral, and some umbilical hernias surgical repair is advised to prevent the risk of strangulation.

Worms

These cause anxiety that is out of all proportion to their clinical importance, as they do not cause any serious problem even if present in large numbers.

Thread, or pin, worms are the main infestation in Britain and the USA and they are present in up to 40% of children below the age of 10 years. Their main symptom is an itchy bottom, especially at night, when the female worms come out to lay their eggs (about 10–15000 for each worm, after which they die). Scratching transfers eggs to fingers, sheets, toilet seats, etc. and onto others' fingers and from there into mouths, starting off the whole cycle again. All members of a family tend to be infected and require treatment even if they have no symptoms.

The adult worms live for only 6 weeks, so if reinfection can be stopped for 6–8 weeks they will all die and the family will be clear. Antiworm medicines, e.g. Pripsen and Vermox, will not be effective alone; sensible hygiene must also be instituted (see Table 12.3).

Table 12.3   Thread (pin) worms — rules of hygiene

Rules (used for 6 weeks)
Affected child Keep nails short. Wear pyjamas and possibly gloves to bed. Bathe each morning and thoroughly wash bottom to remove eggs deposited during the night. Have own towel for sole use. Change and wash clothes and bedclothes. Hoover and dust room thoroughly.
Whole family Fingers and fingernails washed and scrubbed with a nail brush after each visit to the toilet and before each meal. Disinfect toilet seat, door handle, etc.

Piles (haemorrhoids)

These are swellings of the veins on the inside of the anus. They can be related to ageing, constipation, low-fibre diets, and sedentary occupations. Symptoms include itching and soreness of the bottom and spattering of fresh blood on the toilet paper after bowel motions. If the piles prolapse (protrude) then pain may be more severe.

Treatment first consists of a high-fibre diet and avoidance of constipation, with soothing ointments or suppositories to help relieve irritation.

If piles continue to prolapse then injection or operation may be needed. Injection causes shrinking of the piles. Operation is for removal of the piles and is reserved for those that are more troublesome.

Anyone developing symptoms of 'piles' for the first time in middle age or beyond should not assume that the rectal bleeding, pain, or constipation are due to piles. There may be other more serious causes; these have to be checked for by a physician.

Risks and actions
Following commonsense rules of living can help decrease your chances of suffering from gastrointestinal disease.

(1). Brush teeth and gums daily. Avoid sweet foods late at night. This helps to keep teeth and gums healthy to chew food properly and start the digestive process correctly.

(2). Wash hands carefully after going to the toilet and before each meal to ensure you do not pass large numbers of bacteria and viruses onto your food and then into your body.

(3). Cook food carefully. Thaw items from the freezer thoroughly before cooking and do not refreeze. If reheating food be very careful to cook again properly. All these measures are designed to kill bacteria and viruses within food and so cut down your chances of getting food poisoning.

(4). Eat a high roughage diet always (see Appendix 3: Diet for healthy living), as it will keep your bowel motions soft and regular and decrease your chances of developing many bowel diseases from piles to cancer.

(5). If you are overweight — DIET.

(6). If you smoke — STOP.

(7). Do not drink alcohol to excess as liver damage leading to cirrhosis may occur, as may an unnoticed decline into alcoholism.

13
Cardiovascular diseases

Diseases of the heart and blood vessels develop as people age. As we are living longer they have become more prominent causes of illness and death. Heart attacks, strokes, and high blood pressure now cause one half of all deaths in developed countries and are responsible for

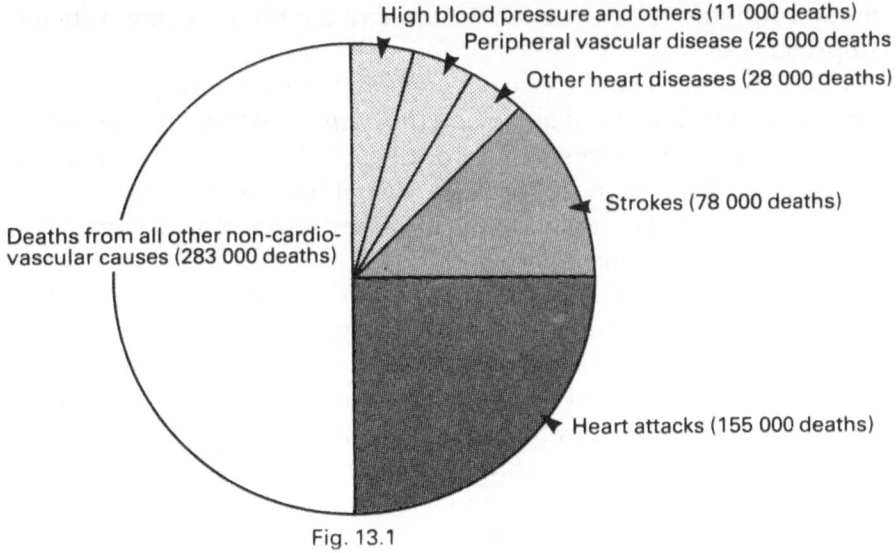

High blood pressure and others (11 000 deaths)
Peripheral vascular disease (26 000 deaths
Other heart diseases (28 000 deaths)
Strokes (78 000 deaths)
Deaths from all other non-cardio-vascular causes (283 000 deaths)
Heart attacks (155 000 deaths)
Fig. 13.1
All cardiovascular deaths (300 000 deaths)

Figure 13.1   Causes of death in England and Wales, 1975.

one in ten of all hospital admissions and for a considerable amount of invalidity and sickness absence from work.

Heart attacks have reached epidemic proportions and strike down active men and women during their working lives. In those who do not die there is a high rate of disability. Although some of the increased numbers of heart attacks are because we live longer and so are liable to this disease of ageing, other causes are the self-inflicted, unhealthy habits of modern living. Overweight, smoking, and taking little exercise may increase the development of atheroma or hardening of the arteries, which then become narrowed or blocked, cutting off the blood supply to vital organs, such as the heart, brain and kidneys. Control of this serious epidemic lies in prevention by healthier personal habits (see page 189), rather than by more and better medical technology to treat the end-results of self-inflicted disease.

Structure and function

By 7 weeks of life in the womb the fetus has a fully developed *heart* which is beating at more than 140 beats per minute. This muscular pump continues to operate day in and day out for a lifetime. When it stops, so ends life.

In an adult the heart beats an average 70 times a minute, moving an average of 80 ml of blood out round the body each time. In a minute it pumps 5.5 l and if under stress, or during exercise, this can increase to 25 or even 35 l. In a 70-year lifetime it moves 202 356 000 l (or 44 968 000 gallons) of blood, at the lowest estimate. An amazing work load for a muscle weighing only 280 g.

Apart from a working heart, a system of patent pipes is needed to carry blood to all parts of the body to supply tissues with food and oxygen. *Arteries* take the fresh blood out from the lungs and heart and the *veins* bring the used blood back (Figure 13.2). The pressure of blood needed at all times to stop the artery walls from collapsing is called the *diastolic blood pressure* and the increased pressure produced as each heartbeat pumps blood into the system is called the *systolic blood pressure*. These two pressures form the 'blood pressure' as measured by the sphygmomanometer.

A useful way of visualizing blood pressure is to consider a garden hose. With no water (pressure) in it it is collapsed; with a steady trickle

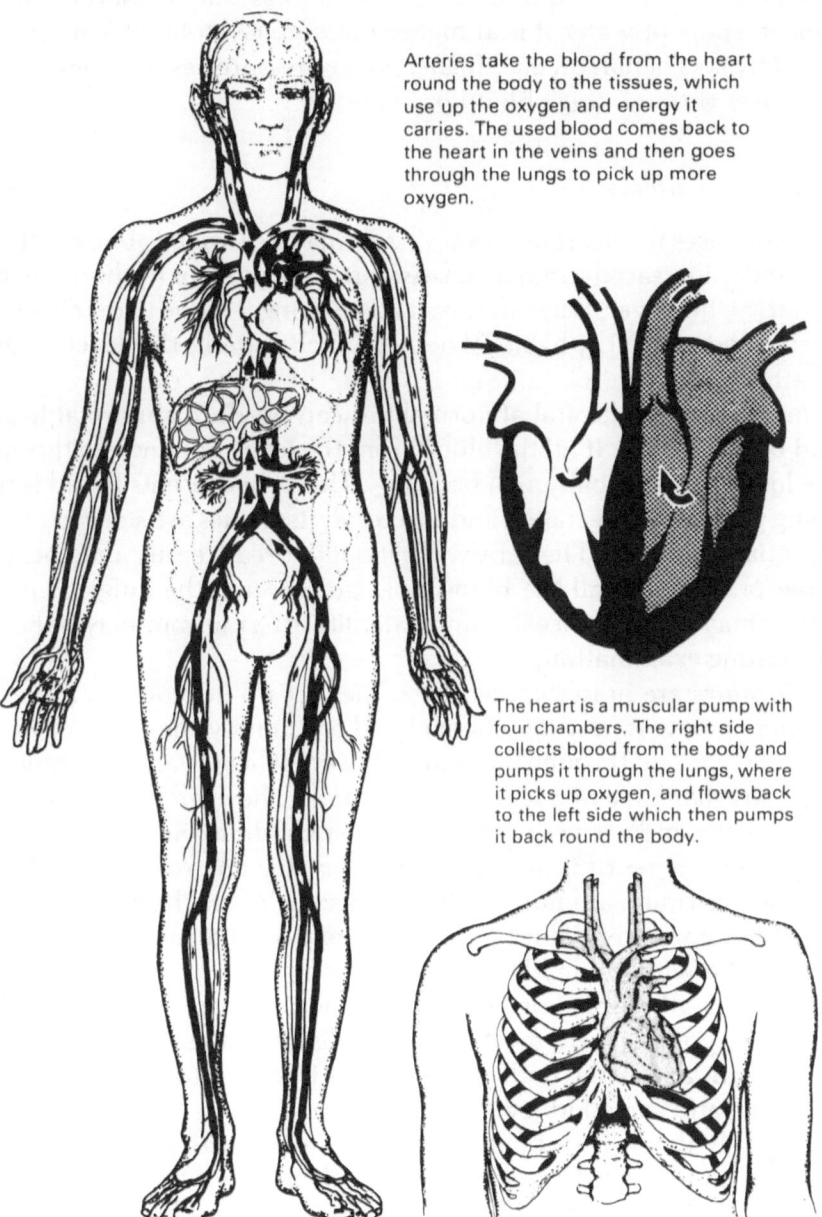

Arteries take the blood from the heart round the body to the tissues, which use up the oxygen and energy it carries. The used blood comes back to the heart in the veins and then goes through the lungs to pick up more oxygen.

The heart is a muscular pump with four chambers. The right side collects blood from the body and pumps it through the lungs, where it picks up oxygen, and flows back to the left side which then pumps it back round the body.

Figure 13.2 The heart and circulation.

of water it is open and at a low pressure (diastolic pressure); with a sudden spurt of water it is at higher pressure (systolic pressure); and with any sort of narrowing a higher water pressure has to be built up to get water through (high blood pressure).

Causes and effects

In some cases the heart or blood vessels may be formed abnormally or put under increased strain by diseases in other parts of the body. In the majority, however, when the heart goes wrong it is due to the effects of ageing and unhealthy habits of living, which underlie the development of atheroma.

In children congenital abnormalities can produce abnormal hearts and blood vessels. If all the blood from the heart does not go through the lungs then the baby will be 'blue'. This is because its blood is not being properly oxygenated and as a result its tissues are starved of this essential substance. The baby will get out of breath easily and does not grow properly. If all the blood does go through the lungs then the effects may not be noticeable until later life, or a murmur may be heard on routine examination.

Murmurs are noises caused by eddies set up in blood as it passes from a narrow to a wider channel and are mainly the result of rapid passage of blood through the heart, abnormal heart valves, or holes in the heart that have no valves to close them. They can be heard with a stethoscope and are very common. Most children will develop one if they have a fever or if their heart goes fast for any reason.

Most murmurs are not due to any disease of the heart. Any child who has an innocent murmur is completely normal and should lead a normal life without any kind of restriction.

In adults atheroma (also known as atherosclerosis or hardening of the arteries) is by far the most important disorder affecting the circulatory system and is the underlying cause of heart attacks, strokes, leg gangrene and some kidney failure.

Basically it consists of patchy fatty deposits being laid down in the walls of middle-sized and large arteries throughout the body. Subsequently these deposits harden and form plaques which extend and multiply, narrowing the arteries and then either blocking them altogether or weakening their walls.

Although fatty streaks can be present in the artery walls of young children, harder atheroma plaques do not appear until early adult life and most of their serious effects not until middle age or beyond.

Severe local narrowing or blockage may cut off the blood supply to heart muscle (producing angina or a heart attack) or to the brain (producing a stroke); this is just a local effect and the atheroma may well be generalized, affecting many arteries throughout the body. The risk factors for developing atheroma are shown in Table 13.1.

Table 13.1 Risk factors for the development of atheroma

High blood fat concentrations	Family history of deaths from heart disease or fat deposits around the eyes or a pale ring around the pupil may suggest this so blood fat concentrations can be measured.
High blood pressure	Untreated high blood pressure is the main cause of strokes. Also causes heart attacks and heart failure.
Cigarette smoking	Most important factor under the individual's control. Increases risk of heart attacks, angina, and poor leg circulation.
Obesity	Only fairly gross levels appear to matter.
Diabetes	Diabetics are at great risk of developing atheroma, especially if they have poor sugar control.
Family history	Important but as likely to be due to similar eating and smoking habits as to genetic factors.
Physical exercise	Leisure exercise protects against heart attacks, which are less likely to be fatal than in those who take no exercise.
Personality	Aggressive, competitive men (type A personality) who are always setting themselves deadlines are at increased risk.

Diseases

Atheroma-related

Angina

This is caused by narrowing of the arteries, reducing blood supply to the heart muscle so that when it needs to work harder its blood and oxygen supply cannot increase enough to meet its needs. This causes a heavy frontal chest pain which may intensify with increased effort, emotion or cold temperature and which clears after a few minutes' rest. Many angina sufferers find that pain is worse in the morning. The course of angina is unpredictable and in many patients it remains mild or ceases altogether. Very few become severely disabled.

It is helped by avoiding situations which may cause the pain; losing weight; stopping smoking; and the taking of tablets of trinitrin (glyceryl trinitrate) which are most effective when put under the tongue *before* doing something which may bring on pain. Trinitrin acts by dilating or opening up arteries. This lowers the blood pressure and so decreases the work the heart muscle has to do, thus relieving the pain of angina. Unfortunately, facial flushing and headaches may be side effects. There are other effective drugs for angina such as beta-blockers (which block certain nerve impulses to the heart and so slow it down) and others that allow the heart to function better. In some severe cases surgical replacement of blocked coronary arteries by leg vein grafts is dramatically successful in relieving the angina.

Heart attacks
These are a major cause of sudden and unexpected death, and are caused by a sudden complete blockage of one of the coronary arteries of the heart resulting in severe damage to the heart muscle fed by that artery.

Attacks can be painless, though usually there is severe, crushing central chest pain which can last for more than 30 minutes. This pain is caused by the damaged heart muscle and may extend into the jaw, into the back, or down the arms. There is often associated sweating, nausea and vomiting, and panic.

If much heart muscle is damaged then the pump action fails and fluid builds up in the lungs, causing severe breathlessness, rapid breathing and, possibly, coughing up of blood-flecked spit. Other complications like shock, abnormal heart rhythm, or even rupture of the heart may occur and about 25% of victims can die in the first few hours.

First aid treatment and immediate intensive care aim to save victims from sudden potentially fatal complications. Irregular heart contractions can be controlled by electric shock treatment to the chest and by drugs. Oxygen helps to reduce the load on the damaged heart.

After a heart attack the aim is to return to normal as soon as possible but with a healthier living programme to try to prevent recurrences and improve general health.

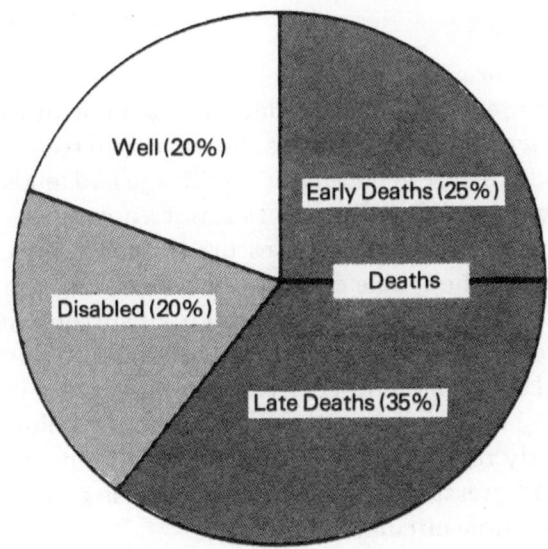

Well (20%)

Early Deaths (25%)

Deaths

Disabled (20%)

Late Deaths (35%)

Figure 13.3   Outcome of coronary artery atherosclerosis.

Heart failure
This results from an inability of the heart muscle to function effectively to pump the blood round the body. A damming-back effect causes fluid to build up in other parts of the body.

Heart failure may occur suddenly after a heart attack or from severe high blood pressure but is more often a more gradual effect of ageing, of chronic bronchitis, or of heart strain from long-standing weakening of the heart muscle from atheroma or raised blood pressure.

In this situation fluid is retained in the body and causes swelling, especially of the feet and legs and breathlessness becomes troublesome.

Diuretic tablets and digitalis (foxglove) are the main drugs likely to be used and they act by increasing the amount of fluid removed from the body by the kidneys, either directly, in the case of diuretics, or indirectly by causing the heart to pump more effectively, as for digitalis. Major changes in life style may be needed to avoid further strain on the heart. More rest, dieting, not smoking, cutting down salt in food, and avoiding stress may help and many with heart failure live into old age.

High blood pressure
This may be caused by kidney or glandular trouble or by drugs (e.g. the contraceptive pill). In most cases, however, no recognizable cause is found. Blood pressure generally rises with age and tends to be higher in men than women. Why this occurs is not known.

The significance of high blood pressure is that, if untreated, it puts greater stresses on the whole circulatory system and can cause some blood vessels to rupture, giving destruction of surrounding tissues. It can also add to heart strain, because the heart has to pump harder to push the blood through blood vessels under higher tension. It can lead to heart attacks, heart failure, strokes, and kidney failure. Successful treatment greatly reduces the risk of these conditions, since reducing the raised blood pressure to nearer normal levels greatly reduces the stresses on the whole circulatory system.

Persons with high blood pressure generally have no symptoms and feel perfectly well and may not see the reason for accepting lifelong care. Headaches, dizziness, etc. come more from worrying about blood pressure once people are told that it is high.

Peripheral vascular disease (claudication)
This is a narrowing of the arteries to the leg muscles giving pain on walking, as the muscle's oxygen needs outstrip the available supply, (like angina). Smoking is a crucial causative factor. By-passes — grafted vessels — can now sometimes be surgically fitted.

Atheroma-unrelated

Palpitations
Sudden changes in the rhythm of the heartbeat will often be felt only as the heart 'beating irregularly' or 'missing a beat', though sometimes they may cause very unpleasant sensations in the chest and fainting attacks.

Feelings that the heart is thumping or missing a beat are very common and most people will have them at some time in their life. They are most often noticed when lying in bed at night and they will disappear with exercise. Most are transient and of no significance. They are normal abnormalities and may be brought on by over-indulgence in tobacco, coffee or alcohol, tiredness, worries or illnesses with a high fever.

Palpitations in young persons are unlikely to be of significance. However, if they occur, for the first time in middle age; if they cause a feeling of faintness or actual fainting; or if they occur in someone who is known to have heart disease, then they must be investigated. They may then be a sign of a serious abnormality of heart rhythm which may need drug treatment (like digitalis) or even an implanted cardiac pacemaker to take over the heartbeat and make it regular.

Varicose veins

These affect almost two out of three adults, most of whom are not bothered by them. Although there are many possible causes only past pregnancy, a family history of varicose veins, and a history of thrombosis of the legs seem to be relevant.

Walking, putting the feet up when resting, and wearing support stockings will help aching veins. Injections into the veins will help most to shrivel for about five years or so, after which the veins tend to recur. An operation to remove the veins altogether may be possible but is only worth considering if the veins really are troublesome, as the results are not perfect.

Deep-vein thrombosis

This occurs in the veins of the leg and is caused by clotting of the blood. Any situation leading to stagnation of the blood in the legs can pre-dispose to this condition, e.g. pregnancy, and bed rest after an operation. It is dangerous only if a piece of clot breaks off into the bloodstream and gets carried to the lung (pulmonary embolism). Happily this is a very rare occurrence.

With this condition the affected part of the leg (usually the calf) becomes very painful, hot, red, swollen, and tender. Treatment is with drugs like aspirin, which decrease inflammation; or with anticoagulants, which thin the blood and stop more clots from forming.

Anaemia

This occurs when the concentration of haemoglobin (the blood's oxygen carrier) drops below normal. It is not a disease in itself but a sign of some underlying disorder. Most commonly it occurs because of iron deficiency either through chronic blood loss (mainly women aged 20—50 who lose excess blood with their periods); poor iron intake in the diet (mainly infants and old people); or poor iron absorption by the body after stomach operations.

Anaemia is often symptomless, though it may cause pallor, listlessness, tiredness, depression, sore tongue, and breathlessness.

After a blood test to determine the exact type and degree of anaemia present, iron tablets by mouth for months or more are the usual treatment. Rarely, iron injections or even blood transfusions may be needed.

Once anaemia has occurred regular checks of the blood should be carried out for years afterwards.

Table 13.2   Cardiovascular risk factors and how to reduce the risk

Risk factor	Action
High blood fat concentrations	Go onto a cholesterol-lowering diet, with reduction of calories if you are overweight. This helps in most people.
High blood pressure	Have your blood pressure checked three yearly before the age of 35 and yearly thereafter. If your pressure is high, remember that *treatment is lifelong and life saving.* Co-operate fully with the physician and take your medication even if you feel well.
Cigarette smoking	Stop.
Obesity	Diet.
Physical exercise	Take regular leisure exercise, though if you are middle aged and out of condition seek medical advice first.
Type A personality	You probably cannot alter this but make sure no other risk factors apply to you.

Prevention and health maintenance

No doctor can prevent heart disease or maintain a healthy circulation for a patient. Individuals can and must do it for themselves and for the killing effects of atheroma there is strong evidence that people can protect themselves by altering their life styles. Table 13.2 summarizes suitable courses of action to take.

14

Nervous disorders

Serious disease affecting the nervous system is not common. However, *symptoms* such as headache and dizziness, which often arise from minor functional disorders of the nervous system, are exceedingly common. It is this divergence between the occurrence of symptoms and the rarity of serious disease that accounts for a good deal of the anxiety surrounding this area. Thus, although headaches are almost universal and brain tumours very rare, the association between the two is recognized.

Apart from the ubiquitous headache, the only diseases of the nervous system which the family physician is likely to treat quite often are strokes and epilepsy. He or she will occasionally see persons with multiple sclerosis or Parkinson's disease but only very rarely someone with meningitis or a brain tumour.

Headaches

What are they?

Headache is one of the most common and disabling conditions experienced by mankind. The head is a complex and vitally important structure containing a large variety of tissue almost all of which can give rise to painful stimuli and cause headache.

Pain may arise from the teeth, the sinuses, the eyes, the ears, the skin, the bones and soft tissue of the neck, the blood vessels of the scalp, and the muscles around the scalp and forehead. Surprisingly, perhaps, one of the few tissues in the head which is insensitive to pain is the brain itself, although the membranes surrounding the brain are exquisitely sensitive.

The cause of a pain in the head or face may be quite obvious. A dental abscess, an acute sinus infection, a discharging ear, a painful eye or a stiff and painful neck, perhaps after a 'whiplash' injury in a road-traffic accident, are all relatively common problems. Similarly, a generalized headache associated with a fever at the onset of a cold or influenza also is a common experience. Rarely, a person may be desperately ill with the sudden onset of a brain haemorrhage or meningitis and it will be obvious that urgent medical attention is required. However, headaches of these types will not be dealt with in this chapter. Rather, the very common problem of headaches, usually recurrent, which affect many and which are not so obviously related to underlying disease as those outlined will be discussed.

Who gets them?

Over 90% of the population experience headaches of some kind at some time in their life. Surveys in several countries have shown that it is an almost universal symptom but that, in general, women are affected twice as often as men and young adults more than either children or elderly people.

Four out of five of the population suffer from headache in any year. Of these headaches, one quarter will be one-sided (unilateral) and not associated with other symptoms, one-fifth will be one-sided and associated with nausea and/or vomiting, and one-fifth one-sided with some warning, such as blurring of the vision, and followed by nausea and/or vomiting. The rest of the headaches experienced will be generalized or localized across the forehead, top of the skull, or back of the head (bilateral).

There has been much debate and discussion about the exact definition of these recurrent headaches, in particular which headaches should be labelled 'migraine' and which 'tension headaches'. The classical types of each are not difficult to distinguish but since both conditions may be so variable, and since both may coexist in the same person, it is not surprising that physicians as well as patients are confused by the terminology.

Tension headaches

These are caused by excessive contraction of the muscles which lie on the surface of the skull, and are usually experienced as a sensation of pressure or heaviness on top of the head or in the forehead. They tend to last longer and be more persistent than migraine attacks and may occur day after day for weeks or months. There may be obvious associated stress, tension, or depression and in these cases treatment of the underlying problem is required. Otherwise, management consists of explanation, reassurance, conscious relaxation and, if necessary, pain-killing or muscle-relaxing drugs.

The outlook for a person suffering from tension headaches is variable. If the headache has been caused by a well-defined stressful situation which may be resolved, then the chance of the headache disappearing is excellent. If, however, the person concerned is chronically unhappy and tense, in a situation which cannot be changed, then the headaches are likely to recur for many years.

Migraine

This may be defined as a headache which comes at intervals with complete freedom between attacks. The headache may be unilateral or bilateral, preceded by visual disturbance such as flashing lights or zig-zag patterns and accompanied by abdominal symptoms such as loss of appetite, nausea, vomiting, and occasionally diarrhoea. In *children* the abdominal symptoms may occur without a headache at all and the condition can be puzzling unless the characteristic pattern is recognized. This condition is known as 'abdominal migraine' or 'the periodic syndrome'. *Classical migraine* is the name usually applied when the complete collection of visual warning symptoms followed by unilateral headache, nausea, and vomiting is present, whilst *common migraine* is used to describe the partial condition where visual symptoms are absent, the headache may be unilateral or bilateral, but the abdominal symptoms are present. *Cluster headaches* or *migrainous neuralgia* are a rather different form of migraine in which the attacks are grouped together in clusters, often waking the victim in the early morning with pain behind one eye which may become red and watery during the attack. Each episode usually lasts between 20 minutes and two hours.

The various types of migraine are summarized in Table 14.1.

Table 14.1   Types of migraine

Type	Warning signs	Headache	Associated symptoms
Classical migraine	Usually visual	Usually unilateral	Nausea and vomiting
Common migraine	None	Usually unilateral	Often nausea and vomiting
Cluster headaches	None	Usually behind one eye	Red and watery eyes
Abdominal migraine (in children)	None	None	Recurrent abdominal pain, vomiting

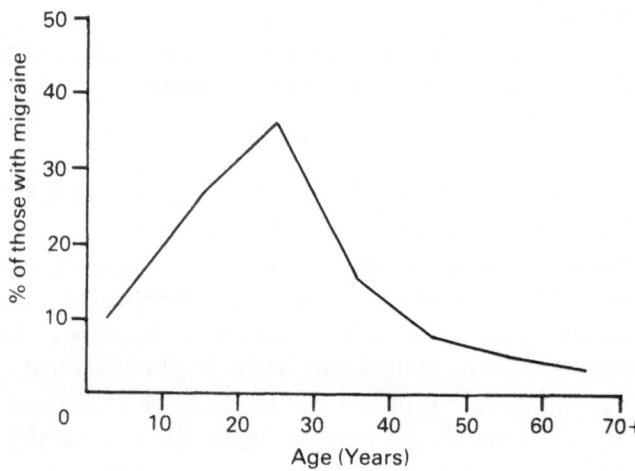

Figure 14.1   Proportion of migraine sufferers at age of onset.

The most common age of onset for migraine is in the teens and early twenties (see Figure 14.1).

At any time only 10% of migraine victims will be disabled with severe and frequent attacks, 30% will suffer an attack at least monthly, whilst 60% will be only slightly inconvenienced by occasional attacks.

There is a definite tendency to improvement with age and after the menopause migraine attacks usually lessen and may disappear altogether.

The cause of the migraine headache is thought to be the over-sensitive nature of the intracranial arteries in susceptible people. In the presence of certain trigger factors the arteries react by constricting excessively, giving rise to the prodromal visual symptoms, and then by dilating excessively and stretching the sensitive nerve fibres in the vessel walls, causing the headache itself. With this model it is possible to see how a logical approach to the prevention, management, and treatment of migraine may be implemented.

The range of possible 'trigger factors' in migraine is very wide and these are listed in Table 14.2.

Table 14.2   Trigger factors in migraine

Anxiety	Fatigue	Travel	Food and drugs:
Worry	Stooping	Climate	Chocolate
Emotion	Lifting	Sunshine	Citrus fruits
Depression	Late-rising	Glare	Cheese
Shock	Fasting	Visual strain	Pastry
Excitement	Dieting	Noise	Fried food
Change of routine		Smells	Alcohol
			Sleeping tablets
			Oral contraceptives

Prevention of attacks

It is important for the migraine sufferer to become aware of the particular trigger factors which seem to be significant in his or her case. It is useful to keep a diary of the timing of any migraine attack and to write down events occurring in the previous 24 hours. In many cases a definite pattern will emerge. The headaches may occur only after eating chocolate or only after lying in on a Sunday morning, having consumed some alcohol the night before. A missed meal may provide the trigger, or excessive stress at work. If particular foods or drinks provoke an attack they can usually be avoided easily but if the problems are caused by the victim's personality, circumstances, or life style then it is likely to be much more difficult to modify these factors.

Treatment of attacks
Whilst prevention is the ideal, there will be many instances where this is not totally successful and it is important that each sufferer should be able to recognize the particular pattern of his or her own attacks. It is a cardinal rule in migraine that the earlier an attack is treated the more likely it is that treatment will be successful and the attack shortened or modified. Whenever possible the sufferer, on recognizing the pro-dromal symptoms, should endeavour to find a quiet, darkened room where he or she can lie down and take the usual medication. In mild cases avoidance of trigger factors, prompt recognition of the problem, rest, and a mild pain-killer such as *paracetamol* or *aspirin* will enable the individual to manage his or her own migraine without recourse to professional help.

Role of the physician
However, there will inevitably also be many patients who either fail to recognize the nature of the condition or who are unable to manage the problem by themselves. The role of the physician is to confirm the diagnosis of migraine and to exclude serious disease. He will usually be able to do this by taking a careful history and conducting a brief examination. It is rarely necessary for any special investigations. The majority can be helped by careful attention to the details already dis-cussed and by using a few drugs which are of special value in migraine.

Use of drugs
Apart from pain-relieving drugs, which have already been mentioned in relation to self-treatment, the physician may prescribe drugs such as *metoclopramide* or *prochlorperazine* which are effective in reducing the associated nausea and vomiting, or possibly a tranquillizer and muscle relaxant such as *diazepam*. However, the drug which is specific for the control of a migraine attack is *ergotamine*. This drug acts by preventing the excessive dilatation of the cranial arteries which is thought to cause the headache and is therefore effective only if administered early in the attack. It may be given in the form of tablets, suppositories, inhalers, or injections and is often dramatically effec-tive. However, the timing and dosage is critical since if taken to excess ergotamine may itself cause nausea, vomiting, and even a headache!
    For those who suffer severe, repeated attacks of migraine, or who

are unable to treat an attack early because they usually wake up with the headache already established, it is sometimes necessary to use preventive treatment. *Clonidine* is a safe drug which can be helpful in perhaps 30—50% of cases and *propranolol*, a so-called beta-blocker, is also useful in migraine. Interestingly, both these drugs were originally introduced for the treatment of vascular diseases such as hypertension and angina before their usefulness in the prevention of migraine was discovered. They are thought to work by diminishing the sensitivity of the blood vessels.

Table 14.3   Useful drugs in migraine

Drug	Effect
Aspirin	Relieves headache
Paracetamol	Relieves headache
Metoclopramide	Relieves nausea
Prochlorperazine	Relieves nausea
Ergotamine	Relieves migraine specifically
Clonidine	Prevents migraine in 30—50% of cases
Propranolol	Prevents migraine in over 50% of cases

Epilepsy

What is it?

We are all potential epileptics. Each one of us, if our brain is stimulated or injured in some way, is capable of suffering the effects of incoordinated abnormal discharges from our brain cells resulting in disturbances of consciousness, of feeling, or of movement — a fit.

The fit may be caused by many agents, including infection as in meningitis, haemorrhage, brain tumour, and high fever particularly in children; disorders of body chemistry; some drugs; and, of course, brain injury from trauma. However, the precise underlying cause of most cases of chronic epilepsy often remains unexplained.

Nevertheless, despite the universal predilection of mankind to this malady, it is a condition which has, since biblical times, been regarded with awe and superstition. It has been regarded as a sign of great spiritual power and holiness, or conversely, a person with epilepsy may be regarded as someone of inevitably low intelligence, prone to inexplicable fits of temper, and disturbing or even dangerous to themselves and others.

Who gets it?

Probably one person in twenty suffers a fit of some sort in their lifetime but only one in eight of those who have a fit will suffer from true epilepsy with a liability to recurrent fits.

Attacks show a progressive decline in frequency with age, and the younger the person on suffering their first attack the better the outlook.

Types of epilepsy

There are different types of epilepsy and some persons may experience a variety of attacks at different times. The most common type is the *febrile convulsion of small children* and other well-defined varieties include *grand mal, petit mal, focal epilepsy,* and *temporal-lobe epilepsy* (see Table 14.4).

Table 14.4   Types of epilepsy

Type	Age at onset	Features
Febrile convulsions	Under 4 years	Grand mal fit associated with fever
Grand mal	Usually under 20 years	Aura, Tonic and clonic convulsions
Petit mal	Childhood	Brief absences without falling or convulsions
Focal epilepsy	Any age	Attacks start in a localized area
Temporal-lobe epilepsy	Usually under 20 years	Unusual aura, Automatic behaviour patterns

Febrile convulsions

This is a common condition of early childhood, affecting possibly one in twenty children, in which a rising body temperature, usually with an infection of the ears or upper respiratory tract, triggers off a classical epileptic fit of grand mal type (see below). Although the condition is alarming to the parents it is normally short lived and does not lead to any permanent damage. Medical advice should be sought, however, so that treatment may be instituted promptly and further investigation arranged if required. The most important preventive action is to take steps to reduce the temperature in any susceptible child by sponging with tepid water and by giving the appropriate dose of aspirin or paracetamol. The outlook is very good (see Figure 14.2) in that 95% of children who have one or more convulsions will have no further attacks after the age of 5 years, i.e. they outgrow them and it does *not* lead to c

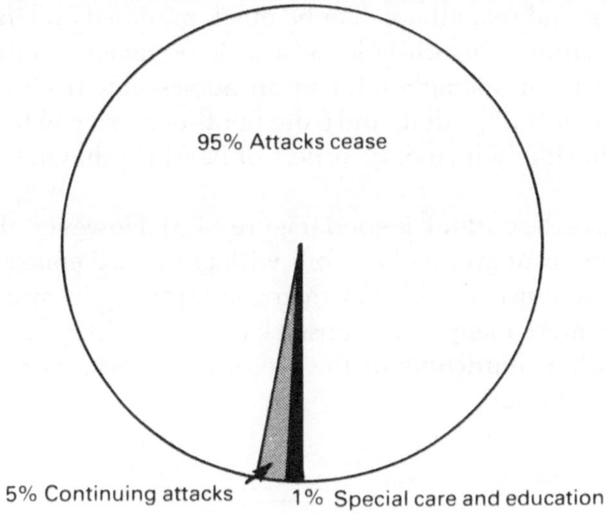

95% Attacks cease

5% Continuing attacks   1% Special care and education

Figure 14.2   Outcome of epilepsy in children.

Figure 14.2   Outcome of epilepsy in children.

Grand mal (major epilepsy)

This is the condition which most people think of as 'epilepsy'. Characteristically, the attack starts with some sort of warning that the fit is about to occur. This is called the *aura*. It may take the form of a general feeling of malaise, an unusual smell or taste, vague abdominal discomfort, or some visual abnormality. The victim may cry out before he or she falls down, the muscles become rigid — the *tonic phase* — and then the limbs move in convulsive jerks for a few seconds — the *clonic phase*. During this stage, he or she may froth at the mouth, bite the tongue and pass urine involuntarily. After the fit the person usually enters a semicomatose state which passes into normal sleep, but occasionally he or she may perform a series of actions automatically without being conscious of what he or she is doing. This is known as *post-epileptic automatism*.

Diagnosis of the condition is apparently relatively easy, and indeed it is in the classic case. However, it can be very difficult because the physician is rarely present at the time of the attack, the victim may not remember it, and witnesses may give a confusing account. In addition, the classical grand mal attack may be much modified and difficult to differentiate from a breath-holding attack or temper tantrum in a young child, from a simple faint in an adolescent, from hysterical convulsions in a young adult, and from faints occurring with cough or micturition in elderly men or disorders of heart rhythm in the elderly of both sexes.

In most cases the outlook is good (Figure 14.3). However, there are a small but significant group of persons with grand mal epilepsy, about 5%, who are seriously disabled by their condition. Epilepsy coming on in later life is more likely to be caused by some underlying structural condition such as hardening of the arteries or pressure on the brain from cysts or tumours.

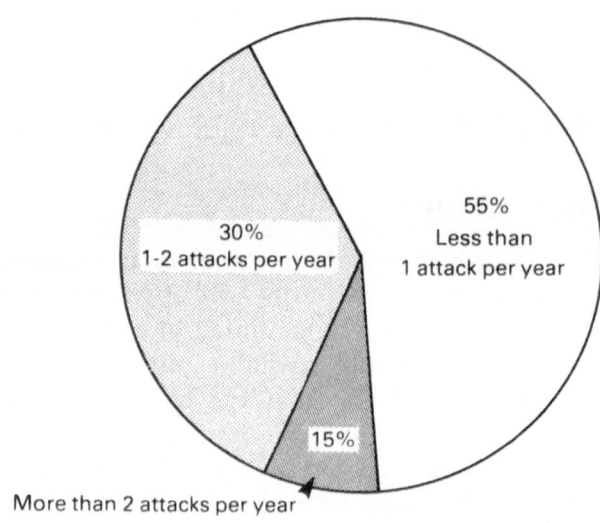

Figure 14.3   Frequency of epilepsy in adults.

Petit mal (minor epilepsy)

This very different form of epilepsy exists only in children. It is characterized by very transitory episodes of loss of consciousness, normally lasting only a few seconds and ending as abruptly as they begin. These blank spells may be so brief as to pass almost unnoticed, since the child will continue a sentence or a drawing without any hesitation. However, since the attacks may occur hundreds of times a day they may affect educational and emotional development. Petit mal can be confirmed by a characteristic pattern in the electrical brain wave scan (electroencephalogram (EEG)).

Petit mal accounts for about 10% of all cases of epilepsy. The attacks may be reduced or abolished by treatment with drugs and as the child grows older the attacks diminish and disappear, although in a few they may be replaced by grand mal, temporal-lobe, or other types of seizure.

Local epilepsy

In this condition the attack starts with involuntary jerking of a localized area, perhaps the thumb or great toe, and gradually spreads to other areas of the body. It may also start as a sensation of localized tingling, coldness, or pain. It is more likely than the other forms of epilepsy to indicate a specific abnormality such as a patch of localized degeneration of brain tissue or pressure.

Temporal-lobe epilepsy

This is a special but relatively common form of focal fit in which the aura often consists of discomfort in the stomach associated with hallucinations of strange sights, sounds, or smells and unpleasant, frightening emotional disturbances. These sensations may precede a major fit or alternatively, a state of automatic action and movement. (The temporal lobe is a certain part of the brain.)

Diagnosis of epilepsy

As can be seen from Figures 14.2 and 14.3 the outlook for children with epilepsy is excellent, whilst in most adults the attacks can be controlled more or less completely with modern drugs. However, a diagnosis of epilepsy is a serious matter because of the profound implications it holds for a patient's life style, and most family physicians would seek a second opinion from a neurologist before making a definite diagnosis. Whilst the diagnosis is usually made on the history of the attacks, it is also usual to undertake some routine investigations, including blood tests, X-rays, and an EEG, to exclude any underlying cause of the attacks which might be surgically treatable. In most cases, no abnormality will be found.

Management of epilepsy

Except for the few cases in which *surgical treatment* is possible to remove diseased brain tissues, the mainstay of management of epilepsy is appropriate *drug therapy*. There is a large and increasing array of drugs available for use in the various forms of epilepsy and it is the responsibility of the physician to choose the most suitable drug or drugs in the appropriate dose so that the person may be kept free of fits without experiencing intolerable side effects. It is now possible to monitor the concentrations of most of the drugs in the blood and this gives more precision in control of therapy. *Phenobarbitone*, for many

Table 14.5   Useful drugs in the management of epilepsy

Drug	Used in	Major side effects
Clonazepam	Grand mal	Drowsiness
Phenobarbitone	Grand mal	Drowsiness, lack of concentration, irritability in children.
Phenytoin	Grand mal	Swollen gums, rash, anaemia, unsteadiness.
Sodium valproate	Grand mal, petit mal, temporal-lobe epilepsy	Nausea, drowsiness.
Primidone	Grand mal	Drowsiness
Ethosuximide	Petit mal	Nausea, drowsiness.
Carbamazepine	Temporal-lobe epilepsy	Rash, anaemia.

years the standard anticonvulsant drug, is now losing some popularity, as also is *phenytoin*, whilst newer preparations such as *sodium valproate* are used more often. However, this is a very complex field in which personal experience of both physician and patient plays a large part in determining the precise dosage and times of medication.

Way of life

There is much more to the control and management of epilepsy than drug therapy alone. The individual patient and his or her physician should be aware of any factors which may precipitate attacks. In febrile convulsions a rapid rise in temperature is the precipitating factor, but in other cases it may be emotional stress, a flickering light or television screen, or an excess of alcohol. The most common reason for a fit occurring in a person who is normally well controlled is that he or she has forgotten or omitted to take the regular medication. It must be very tempting for someone who has not had a fit for years to regard himself or herself as cured and to discontinue medication. This step should not be taken without due consultation with the physician. In particular, suddenly stopping, rather than gradual withdrawal, of a regular drug may provoke a fit. Since this may have profound implications on important matters such as driving a car, employment, or marriage the decision should be carefully considered.

Driving and jobs

Laws do not permit anyone to drive a private vehicle if he or she has had a fit, except during sleep, within the preceding three years. No one may drive a public service or heavy goods vehicle with even a remote history of epilepsy. The diabetic taking insulin is at similar risk. Generally speaking, the same common-sense rules apply to employment. It is obviously unwise for a person with epilepsy to work at heights or with dangerous machinery which cannot be properly screened. Employers tend to be far too rigid in the limitations which they impose on the type of jobs most people with epilepsy can safely perform and it is for this reason that many epileptics conceal their disability. As greater understanding of the condition spreads throughout the general public, employment prospects should improve for the person suffering from epilepsy.

Recreation

Most recreational pursuits are suitable for a person with epilepsy but it is sensible not to swim unaccompanied. There is no reason for a man or woman with epilepsy not to marry and have children but it seems wise that the prospective spouse should be fully informed of all the implications. If two people with epilepsy marry there is a higher risk, about one in eight, that any children of the marriage may themselves become epileptic and for this reason some epileptic couples may decide not to have children.

Strokes

What are they?

A stroke occurs when the functioning of part of the brain is disturbed, either temporarily or permanently, by interference with its blood supply.

The blood supply may be interfered with in a variety of ways. Most commonly, the blood in a damaged artery clots. This is called a *cerebral thrombosis* and accounts for 75% of all strokes. In about 20% one of the intracranial arteries ruptures and a *cerebral haemorrhage* occurs. Less commonly, in 5% or less of cases, a clot from somewhere else in the body, usually the heart valves, moves and lodges in a brain artery and becomes a *cerebral embolus*. In certain cases the brain arteries may go into spasm and produce a *transient ischaemic attack* (TIA).

Significance and outlook

Strokes are becoming more common, since they are essentially a condition of elderly people of both sexes. The average family physician is likely to see 5—8 new cases per year and to be looking after 15—20 people in his or her practice with previous strokes who require continuing care and supervision.

As many as one half of all patients suffering a stroke will die within the first month after the attack. Of the remainder, half will have little or no disability but the other half will be severely disabled. Since the condition is so common in our ageing population, and since such a high proportion of patients will require long-term care and supervision, it is a condition of great economic, as well as personal, significance.

Symptoms

A stroke may present in a variety of ways, ranging from sudden death from a massive cerebral haemorrhage to an episode of transient giddiness or slurring of speech with a TIA. Alternatively, the patient may develop weakness (hemiparesis) or complete paralysis (hemi-plegia) of one side of the body, loss of speech, weakness of a single limb, or visual disturbances. The outlook is better if the victim retains consciousness and if the condition begins to improve within the first few days after the attack.

Management

Where the victim is unconscious or severely disabled he or she will need to be admitted to hospital. In less serious cases, however, the person may fare better at home with support and active rehabilitation. Attendance at a day hospital, rehabilitation unit, or speech therapy centre may be required and persistent help and encouragement may be necessary subsequently.

Prevention

The control and treatment of raised blood pressure is an important preventive measure. Other factors in prevention include giving up smoking and the control of obesity, together with prompt action by the physician if there are any warning signs of an impending stroke. Some patients with cardiac problems take anticoagulant drugs to prevent clots and emboli occurring, and it has recently been suggested that aspirin may have a useful role in the prevention of strokes and heart attacks.

Other neurological disorders

There are many rare conditions which can affect the functioning of the central nervous system. One of these is *multiple sclerosis* (MS), a condition which occurs mainly in younger people in temperate climates and may be due to a very slowly developing virus infection. The characteristic of MS is the extreme variability of the condition, which can present as transient blurring of vision in one eye, weakness of a limb, or abnormal sensations in different parts of the body. Sometimes ten or twenty years may pass between two isolated attacks of the disease with complete remission between attacks. In other cases the condition can deteriorate more rapidly and intensive nursing care and rehabilitation may be necessary. There is no strong evidence that any of the current treatments alter the course or outcome of the disease, although much can be done to make the person more comfortable.

Parkinson's disease (or *paralysis agitans*) is a disease of ageing in which degeneration of a specific area of the brain causes slowness of movement, stiffness, and tremor in one or more limbs, associated with a fixed facial expression, drooling of saliva, and a characteristic shuffling gait when walking. Drug treatment is quite helpful, especially with the relatively new preparation, L-DOPA, which improves many of the associated symptoms. However, this drug does tend to lose some of its beneficial effect after several years and other drugs may then be helpful.

Dementia

Perhaps the most common neurological condition of all, especially with our increasingly elderly population, is *dementia* (or brain failure). In this condition the nerve cells of the brain gradually die, leading to deterioration of memory, intellectual functioning, control over bodily habits, and the patient's personality, causing great anxiety and hardship to relatives and friends during the long, slow decline and deterioration (see also pages 144 and 210).

15
Emotional problems and mental illness

What are they?

Emotional problems arise when emotional reactions which would be considered normal in other circumstances occur in situations where they are clearly inappropriate or when an appropriate emotional reaction is excessively severe or prolonged.

The term *mental illness* is little used by physicians. It can be applied to the extreme forms of emotional problems, to the rare psychoses such as manic—depressive illness and schizophrenia, and to the intellectual deterioration known as dementia. Physicians usually divide mental illnesses into two broad categories:

neuroses — depression, anxiety, and phobias; and
psychoses — schizophrenia, manic—depressive psychosis, and dementia.

The most important difference between these groups is that someone with a neurotic illness has insight: understands that he or she is ill and that what he or she feels is abnormal, while someone with a psychosis has no insight and believes that his or her symptoms, however bizarre they may seem to others, are real and not part of an illness. In fact, the distinction is often not that clear and there is considerable overlap between the two categories.

207

Anxiety

Fear and aggression are normal reactions necessary to survival. Primitive man had to be able to run from predators and fight for his life or in defence of his family or territory. This response is facilitated by the chemical and physical changes necessary to prepare the body for 'fight or flight'. There is increased production in the body of adrenaline. Bowels and bladder empty, pulse rate and blood pressure rise, pupils dilate, the body's secretions are suppressed and the mouth becomes dry, and muscles tremble in readiness for action. All the senses are intensified so that hearing and vision are more acute and there is a greater awareness of events both within the body and in the surroundings.

This primitive response persists still, although the factors which trigger it are different. Everyone recognizes the dry mouth, palpitations, tremor, diarrhoea and frequency of passing urine associated with exams, interviews, making speeches, or listening for burglars in the night. They are accepted as normal. They cease when the stress is removed.

The *morbidly anxious person* has similar symptoms in situations which are not generally accepted as fearful. He or she may suffer from attacks of fear, or panic, during normal everyday activities and experience some or all of the physical symptoms of fear. For example, this may happen in a lift, in a supermarket, going out of the house, at parties, or at work. If the worrying situation continues or if the anxious person has prolonged periods of anxiety then the symptoms may not disappear and may persist for weeks, months, or years. He or she may have persistent diarrhoea, palpitations, tremor, raised blood pressure and increased awareness of various bodily functions as well as a continuing feeling of fearfulness, unease, exhaustion, and despair.

Depression

Similarly, *depression* is a normal human reaction which sometimes gets out of hand. In primitive man, it was probably protective in times of famine or intense cold. The systems of the body slow up and requirements of food and warmth decrease. Pulse rate slows, bowels are sluggish, appetite and sex drive are depressed, and general levels of interest and activity are reduced. The person's attention is turned wholly inwards and he or she appears self-centred and introverted, caring little for anyone else and perhaps even not caring whether he or she lives or dies.

In modern times, depression is most commonly seen in the reaction to marital problems, unemployment, sickness, or bereavement. The picture is often confused by the addition of symptoms of anxiety which accompany the depression. It is normal to feel depressed in unhappy situations.

Someone with a *depressive illness* is depressed to a greater degree, or for longer, than is appropriate to their situation or with little or no apparent reason.

There is no clear dividing line between normal and abnormal, or excessive, emotional reactions. What is normal for one person is excessive for another. Everyone has to learn to be flexible with themselves and with others when considering emotional problems. This is particularly difficult for people in long-term unhappy situations. It is obviously normal for the wife or husband of an alcoholic to be depressed and anxious; but how severely depressed, and for how long?

It is usual for psychiatrists to divide depressive illness into two types: those which are precipitated by some external event, such as bereavement, and are called *reactive or exogenous depression*; and those which arise for no apparent reason from within the individual — *endogenous depression*. Typically, the symptoms are slightly different. In practice, the division is not at all clear and there is a large, grey area where the two ends of the spectrum overlap and the distinction may be more of a nuisance than a help.

There is a rare and extreme form of endogenous depression characterized by wild swings of mood, which it is useful to distinguish. The sufferer experiences periods of excessive elation, or mania, when he or she is very active, needs little sleep, talks and thinks fast and behaves incongruously, spending lots of money and quarrelling and picking arguments. These alternate with periods of intense depression of the classical endogenous type. The whole condition is known as *manic—depressive psychosis* and is characterized by the lack of insight typical of psychotic illness.

Schizophrenia

Schizophrenia is the term applied to a group of conditions in which normal thought processes are disrupted and the individual experiences sensations, feelings, sights, or sounds, which are not recognized as normal by those around him. His or her interpretation of the behaviour of other people may be abnormal so that relationships deteriorate and he or she may become paranoid. These features do not usually apply to all aspects of behaviour at all times and he or she may sometimes appear completely normal. The most important feature of the condition is a total lack of insight into the abnormal nature of the symptoms. A depressed or anxious person is able to recognize the symptoms as such even if he or she cannot understand or control them. A schizophrenic — whose delusion is that he or she is being watched or controlled by outside forces — believes that this is in fact the case, and may respond accordingly, causing great trouble.

Dementia (or brain failure)

This is a deterioration of intellectual function which develops as a result of disease of the brain. The commonest cause is atherosclerosis ('hardening of the arteries') which occurs in the elderly. In this condition, the blood supply to the brain is reduced and the cells are starved of oxygen.

Range of normal

Without exception, every normal, healthy individual suffers at one time or another from anxiety and depression either together or separately. They may be called worry and sadness but the feelings are the same and the labels unimportant. The terms anxiety state and depressive illness are applied to these feelings when they arise inappropriately or are abnormally intense.

Who gets them and why?

It is impossible to know the exact prevalence of anxiety and depression because they are difficult to define precisely and because most people do not seek medical help for these conditions. It seems likely that about 16% of the population are suffering from a depressive illness at any one time and far more do so at some time in their lives. It occurs at any age and in both sexes. Women are more likely to suffer from depression than men, especially in the postnatal period and during the menopause. It is common in children but often is not recognized.

Those most likely to suffer from depression include women who are socially isolated, have several children under school age, have no work or interest outside the home, or who have difficulty in communicating with their husbands.

There is great variation in susceptibility of individuals to mental illness. It is likely that everyone would eventually suffer mental illness (nervous breakdown) if subjected to sufficiently intense stress. The intensity of stress required to induce the illness and the form of illness produced depend on the personality type and vulnerability of the individual.

Vulnerability depends to a great extent on childhood experience and success in dealing with early problems. The foundations of emotional stability and resistance are laid between birth and 5 years and developed during the succeeding ten years. Serious difficulties during this period impair emotional stability for the future.

Personality type probably depends partly on inherited characteristics and partly on early experiences. At one extreme are those who normally have swings of mood with ups and downs: the sociable extrovert — at some times the life and soul of the party, at others fed up with life. This is known as a cyclothymic personality and under extreme stress such a person is likely to break down in the direction of manic—depressive illness. At the other extreme are those who tend to be naturally withdrawn and introverted, quiet and isolated. They are more likely to break down with a schizophrenic illness, if subjected to intolerable stress. Most people have personality types between these extremes and stress is never so severe for them as to produce breakdown of any sort. However, for those who are particularly vulnerable, no great stress is needed to precipitate a breakdown and in them a depressive illness or anxiety state may develop under the pressures of normal life.

The importance of emotional problems and mental illness lies in the misery they cause for the patient and his or her family and in the disruption to normal family life and subsequent detriment to development of stable personalities in the children. The occurrence of suicide and violence because of mental illness is extremely rare.

What effects?

Depression and anxiety

Apart from the general slowing up of depression and the preparation for 'flight and fight' characteristic of anxiety, both these conditions cause a variety of physical (neurotic) symptoms. These result from the despairing and inward-looking orientation of the depressed person and the increased awareness of bodily functions of the anxious. In addition, people who are depressed often subconsciously feel the need for help and minor physical symptoms like backache and headache, which they might normally ignore, may be magnified into major problems for which help is needed. It should be emphasized that the symptoms are real and not invented or imagined and that the sufferer may not be aware that depression is the underlying cause. Sufferers must never be labelled as 'malingerers'. This is wrong and unfair. Concurrent unhappiness is often thought of as either irrelevant or resulting from the symptom. An anxious person with his or her heightened awareness of bodily functions may sense the heart beating and bowels moving, as well as being worried more than usual about minor physical symptoms. Any of these sensations may become magnified into major problems and the anxiety attributed to the symptom rather than the other way round.

Features of depression
Lethargy — often waking tired.
Lack of interest in work, family, hobbies, or appearance.
Loss of appetite — especially loss of enjoyment of food.
Weight may fall or it may rise due to eating for comfort or because laying down fat is the reaction of some individuals to stress.
Loss of interest in sex.
Sleeping difficulty: persistent waking very early in the morning may be a sign of increasing depressive illness.
Constipation.
Feelings of self-deprecation, self-blame and excessive guilt.

Features of anxiety
Feelings of fear, panic, unease — sinking feeling.
Dry mouth.
Palpitations and faintness.
Diarrhoea.
Frequency of micturition.
Increased sweating.
Clenching of teeth and hands.
Irritability, ill temper.
Sleep disturbance.
Loss of appetite.
Loss of weight.

Features common to both depression and anxiety
Menstrual disturbances.
Insomnia.
Backache.
Headache.
Chest pains.
Phobias — especially fear of cancer and fear of dying.
Digestive disturbances.
Difficulties in personal relationships.
Poor concentration.

What happens?

Of those who suffer from depression, roughly one third have one attack only and recover, one third have repeated attacks, and one third are chronically depressed.

The *outcome* of a particular illness depends more on the personality and emotional resources of the individual and on the amount of family and social support available than on medical treatment. Medical care apparently has little effect on the eventual outcome, although symptoms may be alleviated and the duration of the illness shortened.

Prevention of mental illness is difficult to set up. Common sense is essential if wrong interpretations are to be avoided. Anyone is protected if he or she has had a happy and secure infancy and childhood. If not, then there is little that can be done, later in adult life, to repair the damage. It helps for everyone to understand his own emotional weaknesses and those of his immediate family and to learn to live with and make allowances for them. This is particularly important within marriage and greater understanding of the imperfections of all normal marriages is necessary if problems are to avoided. The honeymoon and early marital bliss are short lived and realities come with the every-day routine of work, living together, and raising a family. Mental illness in the next generation might be prevented if today's young adults had a better understanding of marriage and children before they start a family. Many children are now treated with little understanding and scant respect, and their future emotional stability is uncertain.

What to do

Only about one in five of all who suffer from depression consult a physician about it. Most of those who do need only reassurance and some interpretation of their symptoms. A few may be helped by anti-depressant drugs; less than 10% of those seen by a family physician need referral to a psychiatrist.

Most of the help depressed people receive comes from the immediate family, friends, neighbours, counsellors, church, and social workers. The roles of these helpers are not easy. Feelings of guilt and shame are common in depression and often cause people to try to hide their symptoms even from themselves. Many feel there is a social stigma attached to the illness and that it is due to weakness. This attitude is not helpful. Clearly no one likes being depressed and would 'pull themselves together' if he or she could. He or she does not need to be urged to do so. Too much sympathy can also be counter-productive and remove the drive to recover, which is already weak. A depressed person needs practical help, emotional support and acceptance, and understanding accompanied by a firmly optimistic view of the future outcome of the illness.

Antidepressant drugs are most useful in the endogenous type of depression. They have the effect of lessening the depth of despair and possibly of shortening the total illness. Most of them have a gradual effect, taking between ten days and three weeks to produce any notice-able change. During this time, some side effects may be felt and the patient may be tempted to stop the drug, considering it worse than useless. The side effects usually consist of a dry mouth and drowsiness and may be reduced by taking the bulk of the daily dose at night. They lessen after the first two or three weeks and are not usually a problem after that. It is usual to continue to take the antidepressant drugs for a prolonged period — at least three months — and to reduce them gradually over a further month if a relapse is to be avoided.

Tranquillizers may be useful in reducing the effect of intense anxiety over a short period but they rapidly lose their effect and cannot be usefully continued for more than a few days. One side effect of tranquillizers is to cause depression and they therefore have little place in the treatment of that condition.

Most sleeping tablets (hypnotics) are tranquillizers in larger dose and have the same drawbacks. They do improve disturbed sleep for a few nights but after that the improvement becomes less noticeable, until the old pattern is re-established. If they are taken regularly for more than ten days, then the individual becomes habituated and will find that stopping them causes insomnia worse than the original problem. Their main use is at times of crisis or for people working occasional night shifts who cannot sleep in the day. Even then, they are best avoided.

16

Respiratory diseases

The most common group of human diseases are those affecting the respiratory tract (the breathing apparatus). Figure 16.1 shows that in the community with self-care and in family medical practice respiratory diseases account for one quarter to one third of all conditions, and that they are the third most common cause of death.

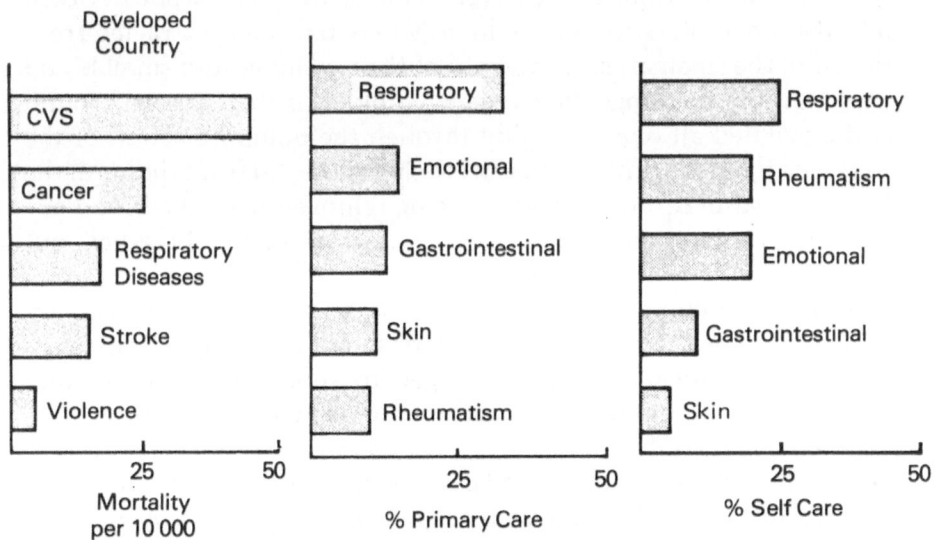

Figure 16.1   Causes of illness and death.

What are they?

In descending order of prevalence they are:

> Acute upper respiratory infections; that is, coughs, colds, flu, sore throats, and infections of ears.
> Acute bronchitis and pneumonia.
> Chronic bronchitis—emphysema.
> Hay fever, other nasal allergies, and sinus problems.
> Asthma.
> Lung cancer.

Although a family physician may expect to see in a typical year 600 or so of his or her patients with common acute upper respiratory and ear infections, 150 with acute bronchitis and pneumonia, 35 with bronchitis—emphysema, and 25 with asthma, he or she will diagnose only one or two new cases of lung cancer in the practice of 2500 persons in a year.

Structure and function of the respiratory tract

The respiratory tract is designed for breathing and the aims of the respiration (the breathing process) are to inhale air, to transport it down into the inner interstices of the lungs where oxygen is extracted from the air in the small air sacs (alveoli) of the two lungs into small blood vessels. From the lungs the oxygenated blood is then carried around and circulated all over the body through the pumping action of the heart. At the same time as oxygen is being extracted from the air in the lungs, so waste carbon dioxide is being removed from the blood circulating the lungs into the air sacs and eventually breathed out (exhaled).

This highly complex biochemical process takes place continually during life. For if we stop breathing for long then the body ceases to function because of a lack of oxygen to supply vital organs and because of an accumulation of carbon dioxide within the body.

To enable these functions to be carried out the respiratory tract is designed to transport the air and gases in and out; to purify, moisten, and warm the air; to remove foreign particles; to destroy noxious germs and other dangerous substances; and to exert a bellows effect to build up sufficient forces for inhalation and exhalation (Figure 16.2).

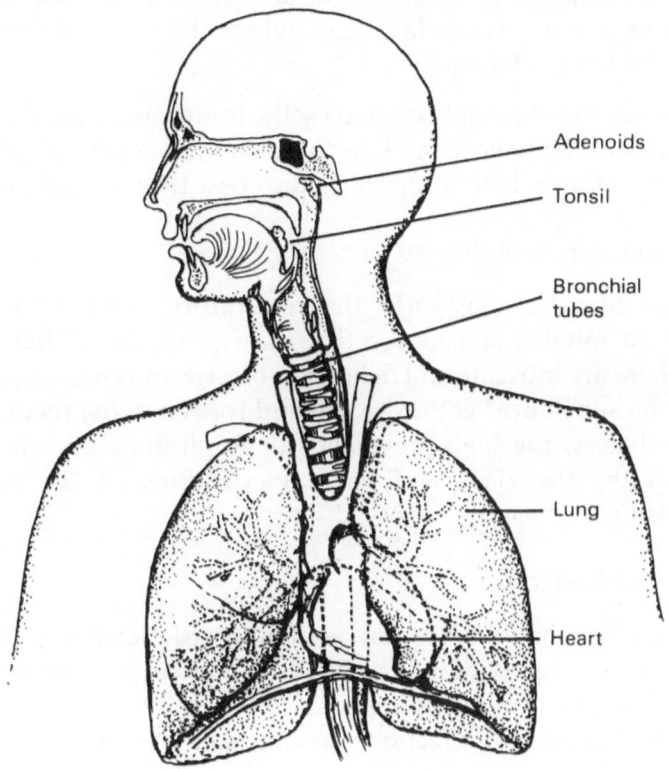

Figure 16.2   The structure of the respiratory tract.

For convenience the respiratory tract can be divided into:

The upper respiratory tract — The nose, mouth, throat and larynx, and the ears which communicate by tubes with the back of the throat. This region cleans and moistens the air in the nose and the larynx as well as being responsible for voice production, and protects the middle and lower regions from food and foreign bodies that may be inhaled if they 'go the wrong way'.

The middle respiratory tract — The windpipe (trachea) and bronchial tubes; these are conducting channels that also help to moisten the inhaled air and to remove the exhaled air.

The lower respiratory tract — The lungs; these include the many millions of minute alveoli (air sacs), where the essential processes of gaseous exchanges take place.

The lungs in the chest are covered by the bony ribs, which are moved by muscles in the bellows action; this also includes the diaphragm or large sheet of muscle that separates the chest from the abdomen.

Causes and effects of disease

Since we breathe constantly the respiratory tract is continually exposed to inhaled substances that may cause harm and damage. Hence there are intricate and delicate protective mechanisms designed to stop the substances getting down and for removing them.

Nevertheless, the high prevalence of respiratory infections noted demonstrates the risks and the imperfections of the protective mechanisms.

Viruses and bacteria

These may be inhaled by contact with infected material usually from other human beings or animals, and some may settle in the respiratory tract, causing clinical infections.

The most prevalent infections are caused by viruses that settle in, and infect, the upper and middle respiratory divisions causing colds, coughs, catarrh, flu, sinusitis, sore throats, and infections of the middle ear.

Pneumonias (infection of the lungs) tended to be caused more often by bacteria than viruses. Most bacteria tend to be stopped and destroyed in the upper respiratory tract and so pneumonias are uncommon, but are more serious conditions when they occur.

Inhaled pollutants and irritants

These, such as from tobacco, dirty air with sulphur and smoke, chemical and organic fumes at some occupations, and of course radioactive substances, may cause serious harm to the lungs and respiratory tract. Tobacco smoke inhaled over 20 years or so can lead to cancer of the bronchi (lung). Cancers may result also from work with some industrial processes and from inhalation of radioactive substances.

Chronic bronchitis and emphysema may be the end-results of years of smoking and inhaling dirty air at work and in the community. The coldness and humidity of the air may also cause damage.

As well as hazards from inhaled substances, lung disorders may be associated with inherited predispositions such as asthma and cystic fibrosis.

Diseases

Common infections

Upper respiratory infections (URI)
These are the coughs and colds that tend to be seasonal and inevitable. Some are more prone to them than others. It seems that children suffer most, and old persons fewest, common colds and coughs. Those who are 'always catching colds' are more likely to be suffering from an oversensitive allergic nasal lining (vasomotor rhinitis) than from infective colds.

The causes of many URI are a wide range of viruses, some known and many unknown. Since they are many and since there are no specific antibiotics for them, there can be no good and effective preventive vaccines nor any antibiotics to use.

Influenza is caused by a specific virus, the influenza virus, that is more virulent than the more usual URI viruses. It has the unfortunate tendency to change its strains and each new strain is really a new virus to which human beings find it difficult to acquire an immunity.

It is because of the virulence of the virus and lack of long-term immunity that influenza is an epidemic condition, often sweeping across countries and continents.

The main features are sudden onset; generalized aches, fever, and cough; and nasal discharge. The acute state lasts for up to a week unless progress is delayed by complications such as bronchitis and pneumonia.

There is no special treatment. Chest complications are treated with antibiotics. Immunization is possible because vaccines can be prepared but benefits are uncertain because of the uncertainty of the likely strain of the infecting virus. It is quite impossible and uneconomical to immunize whole populations with flu vaccines that are uncertain in action and transient in duration.

Bronchitis and pneumonia

These are infections of the bronchial tubes and of the lungs ('pneumonitis' is another term, similar to 'bronchitis', denoting inflammation of the lungs). Although some infections may be caused by viruses, bacteria are more usual causes. Among the causal bacteria are pneumococci, staphylococci, streptococci, and others.

The effects of bronchitis and pneumonia are locally to produce cough with yellow sputum, and considerable malaise and fever. Severe, widespread pneumonia puts considerable areas of the lungs out of action and interferes with the whole process of respiration. In addition the infection may spill over into the bloodstream causing septicaemia (blood poisoning).

Before the availability of antibiotics, pneumonia and bronchitis were not an uncommon cause of death. Now antibiotics control the infection of most types of pneumonia, including tuberculosis, and give the body a good chance to recover.

Chronic bronchitis—emphysema is a confusing condition; despite the word 'bronchitis' it is not a true infection but rather a condition with a mixture of causes and end-results.

The main features are productive cough, an increased liability to acute bronchitis and pneumonia, and slow destruction and obstruction of areas of the lungs and smaller bronchial tubes.

Persons affected may start with a productive 'smoker's' morning cough; they may suffer one or two attacks a year of acute bronchitis with fever and wheezing. Then gradually they begin to experience persisting shortness of breath that may become so severe that going out of doors becomes impossible.

The probable causes are cigarette smoking and living and working in atmospherically polluted areas with damp and cold winters, such as in Britain. In addition there seems to be some hereditary liability in some families.

Once present there is no effective cure. The only hope lies in prevention: by immediately giving up smoking, by treating each attack of acute bronchitis seriously with antibiotics and other measures, and by avoiding inclement weather and hazardous occupations if possible.

Unless preventive steps are taken chronic bronchitis — predominantly a condition of men from middle age onwards — tends to worsen, with increasing disability.

Pulmonary tuberculosis
This is a special type of lung infection caused by the tubercle bacillus, which produces a less acute and more chronic and relentless infection of the lungs.

Asthma
This is another unhelpful term. The usual understanding of 'asthma' is a person suffering from attacks of breathlessness and wheezing. But there are many causes and types of wheezy chests.

The structural changes that lead to bouts of breathlessness and wheezing are transient narrowing of the smaller bronchial tubes. Their diameter may be reduced by more than one half and as air is sucked in and out of the narrowed tubes a wheezy sound is heard by the victim and observers. Because the bronchial tubes are narrowed the amount of air inhaled is reduced and breathlessness results. Because air cannot be expelled easily the chest may become overinflated during severe attacks.

During an attack the victim is short of breath and distressed and there is an accompanying irritating cough. He or she prefers to sit rather than to lie down.

The *chief causes and types* are:

Acute wheezy chests in children — The attacks are part of the 'catarrhal child syndrome' (page 101) and usually are triggered off by a bronchial infection. Almost all (more than nine out of ten) outgrow these attacks by the age of 15 years.

Acute wheezy attacks in chronic bronchitis (see above) — Bouts of wheezing and breathlessness in chronic bronchitics are common. Some are associated with infections but in others the attacks may appear without an obvious infection. Such attacks may lead to further permanent deterioration in the condition.

Wheezy breathlessness — This may rarely be caused by local partial blockage of bronchial tubes from enlarged glands, tumours, or even an inhaled foreign body such as a nut or small toy.

True asthmatic attacks — These occur at intervals and are unrelated to chronic bronchitis or underlying dust diseases. The attacks come on suddenly and often unexpectedly. In susceptible subjects they may be triggered by substances such as dusts, pollens, feathers, hair, exercise, infections; drugs such as aspirin; or foods such as shell fish.

There is often a family history of asthma or other allergies, such as hayfever or eczema.

Specific definable allergies are more likely to be found in asthma that starts in childhood. Asthma starting in adult life tends to be unassociated with allergies.

Whatever the type of asthma there is a tendency for the attacks to improve naturally after a number of years of activity. In my own practice only 5—10% of all asthmatics have become seriously disabled.

The management of asthma is a personal affair. Specific trigger factors must be avoided. The acute attack is managed by drugs that release and relieve the spasm and narrowing of the bronchial tubes. Long-term care may require antiallergic drugs such as Intal (sodium cromoglycate) or one of the corticosteroids. Antibiotics may be necessary for acute infections. Specific desensitization with vaccines have a limited role because their results are unpredictable and there are serious risks to their use.

Cancer of the bronchi (lung)

This is increasingly common. The bronchi are now one of the three most common sites for cancer. The other two are the female breast and the bowels (colon and rectum).

Cancer of the lung arises in the cells lining the bronchi. It is often the consequence of chronic irritation from years of inhaling irritating and hot cigarette smoke. Eventually some of the cells become so irritated that they turn cancerous and grow rapidly in a highly disordered manner and invade adjacent tissues and structures. Some of these disordered cancer cells break off and settle in other parts of the body, forming satellite cancer colonies.

Locally, the cancer produces a tumour within the bronchial tube. This can cause further irritation and cough. It may become eroded and produce expectoration of blood. The bronchial blockage may result in the lung behind the obstruction being put out of action, causing breathlessness, and it may become infected with pneumonia.

Spread of the cancer causes general ill health, loss of weight, weakness, and depression, and local effects may affect the function of organs such as the brain, or cause pain by affecting the spine.

There is no effective treatment for lung cancer. The success rates of surgical removal of the affected lung and tissues, of radiotherapy, or of drugs is less than 10%.

The best management of lung cancer is not to have it. It can nearly always be prevented by not smoking. Once it is there it is too late. It is much better never to start smoking.

Risks and actions

Fortunately, although disorders of the respiratory tract are so common, most are minor ailments that cause much nuisance but few serious effects. They tend to resolve on their own, given time. The best ways of treating them are to give them time to clear and to avoid potent and potentially dangerous drugs.

Acute bronchitis and pneumonia are common but fortunately many attacks are speedily responsive to modern antibiotics.

Asthma is a personal disorder affecting individuals with hypersensitive bronchial tubes that pass into bronchospasm with breathlessness and wheezing for various reasons or for no obvious reason. Here, there are also effective modern preventive and relieving drugs. The natural outlook for asthmatics is good.

The most serious disorders of the respiratory tract are chronic bronchitis—emphysema and cancer of the lung and bronchi. Both are largely preventable. It is clearly established that there is a definite relationship between cigarette smoking and lung cancer and severe, chronic bronchitis.

Preventive actions are entirely in the hands of the individual. The risks of cigarette smoking by now must be known to everyone. Lung cancer can nearly always be avoided and severe chronic bronchitis nearly always prevented by not smoking.

17
Infectious diseases

The term *infectious disease* is an inexact one. It is usually applied to a disease in which the body is invaded by a micro-organism, which can be identified, which causes a distinctive illness, and which can be transmitted to another person. The term is not usually applied to diseases due to parasites, such as worms, mites, or insects, which are known as *infestations*, although these may act as vectors (carriers) of infectious diseases. Nor are *localized infections* such as ringworm, boils, or impetigo usually called infectious diseases.

Micro-organisms causing infectious diseases come from several different groups: viruses, bacteria, rickettsiae, fungi, and protozoa. Some are still not firmly classified. Some, like smallpox, are highly virulent and cause disease in a high proportion of the people who come into contact with them. Others affect only those whose resistance is low and cause no or only very mild illness in normal, healthy subjects.

The *method of transmission* is also varied. Skin infections and venereal diseases are contagious, i.e. are transmitted by touch. Most virus infections are transmitted by droplets of infected material which hang in the air near an infected person. Food poisoning, dysentery, and typhoid develop only after the ingestion of infected material, such as contaminated food or water. Malaria, plague, and typhus are spread by insects, and rabies by animals.

227

Infectious diseases are called *endemic* when they are constantly present. Many infectious diseases also occur in outbreaks, or *epidemics*.

The pattern of infectious disease

This varies in any community from time to time and depends on a number of different factors, some of which are mentioned here.

Climate and local flora and fauna

For example, malaria occurs only in warm, marshy areas where the anopheline mosquito thrives. Schistosomiasis, though strictly an infestation, demonstrates this well, as it relies on an intermediate host, a snail, which is common in Africa, South America, and eastern countries but which does not occur in the UK or USA.

Methods of sewage disposal

Cholera, for example, is usually spread by the contamination of drinking water with sewage and therefore occurs where sewage disposal is inefficient or non-existent or not used by the people.

Culture and life style

Venereal diseases are most common where promiscuity is at a high level. Schistosomiasis is contracted by the penetration of the skin by the parasite swimming in water and so occurs when people spend time with bare feet in water, as when planting rice in a paddy field.

Standards of living

Individual resistance to infectious disease depends upon a high standard of nutrition, housing, education, and adequate clothing and warmth as well as the avoidance of repeated debilitating infections. In addition, some diseases, like tuberculosis, spread most easily when people live in overcrowded conditions. Where standards of hygiene are low, infections spread by contamination of food are common.

Virulence of organisms

This seems to wax and wane so that a disease like scarlet fever, which used to be severe, is now mild.

Immunization programmes

These have had a dramatic effect on some infections, notably small-pox, which has now been eradicated from the world by vaccination. Whilst its importance to individuals cannot be overemphasized, the influence of immunization on the overall incidence of most other infectious diseases has been less dramatic. For instance, diphtheria, tuberculosis, whooping cough, polio, and measles have become less prevalent; but they had all started to decline in western countries, mainly because of the rising standards of living, before the introduction of immunization.

Individual and racial variations

These certainly exist in susceptibility to infectious diseases but are complex. They are made more difficult to study because of social, nutritional, and climatic differences between different communities. An epidemic of measles has a devastating effect and high mortality in an African community but how much of this is caused by individual or racial characteristics and how much by malnutrition and general debility is difficult to say. One intriguing observation is that people who suffer from sickle-cell anaemia, a hereditary blood disease, are less likely to suffer from malaria but have an increased susceptibility to some other infections.

Availability of effective treatment

This is crucial in those diseases, such as tuberculosis, which respond well to treatment with appropriate antibiotics. It is less important in those diseases like rabies and smallpox which are not influenced by treatment. In some, such as measles, the disease itself is not amenable to therapy but the complications are, and in this case antibiotics have transformed the disease from a serious to a relatively minor problem. In some infections, it is the symptoms which endanger life. This is particularly true of gastroenteritis in infants and of cholera; here adequate replacement of fluids and electrolytes is now standard practice and can be life saving.

Prevention of infectious disease

This has to be approached from two angles: that of the community as a whole and that of each individual. In addition, certain diseases need special measures.

Prevention in the community

Most infectious diseases are reduced in incidence and severity by a high standard of living. The most important preventive measures are therefore political and economic. Public health measures are also of great importance:

Maintenance of safe food and water supplies — e.g. by inspection of dairy herds for tuberculosis and brucellosis; of food preparation and packaging centres for standards of hygiene; frequent examination of drinking waters.

Eradication of disease-carrying parasites and their hosts, e.g. bedbugs, lice, and rats.

Investigation of outbreaks and identification of carriers. Many infections are spread by contamination of food by an infected person, either someone suffering from the disease or a symptomless carrier such as the notorious 'typhoid Mary' who worked as a cook and spread the disease widely in North America.

Follow-up of contacts who may be symptomless but infectious.

Immunization programmes including as many as possible of the community.

Prevention in individuals

Prevention is aimed at avoiding infection, minimizing the severity of an attack and avoiding complications, and increasing individual resistance through immunity. In the past, the main method of avoiding infection was by the use of quarantine, or isolation, of people suffering from infectious diseases and their contacts. This never worked well because of the high proportion of very mild cases who are never recognized, but nevertheless are infectious. Many infections are infectious before symptoms appear and isolation is too late to prevent spread. Most schools still operate a system of quarantine and exclude children from school for a specified time for each infectious disease but there is no good justification for this.

Nowadays, immunization is the main weapon used in the prevention of the more serious infectious diseases. Details of immunization procedures are explained in Chapter 5. Malaria is a good example of a disease for which special measures are needed. Attempts are usually made where possible to eradicate the anopheline mosquito and this has been achieved in the UK and USA. Malaria is one of the few diseases which are prevented in those who travel to and live in malarious areas by taking antimalarial drugs before, during, and after their stay. The drugs act by killing any malarial parasites that enter the body from the mosquito bite.

Infectious diseases in the UK and USA

The commonest endemic infectious diseases in the UK, USA and other developed countries are listed in Table 17.1.

Immunity

As a result of an infection with some micro-organisms, the individual develops chemical antibodies which confer lifelong immunity to the disease. This is called *active immunity*. Infants have a *temporary (passive) immunity* from antibodies passed on from the mother during intrauterine life and from breast milk. By about 1 year, the effect of these has worn off and the child is then susceptible. Children contract most of the common infections before their teens, unless they have been immunized. These infections are therefore less common, but tend

Table 17.1 The most common infectious diseases in the UK, USA, and other developed countries

Disease	Cause	Spread by	Incubation period	Infectivity	Immunization If available	Immunization If used	No. consulting a doctor per 1000 population per annum
Mumps (epidemic parotitis)	Virus	Droplets in the air near infected person.	14–21 days (usually 18)	Until swelling has has subsided.	Yes	Yes in USA No in UK	2
Measles (morbilli)	Virus	Droplets in the air near infected person.	10–15 days (usually 10)	From onset until 4 days after appearance of rash.	Yes	Yes	5
Chickenpox (varicella)	Virus (varicella)	Droplets in the air near infected person.	11–21 days (usually 14)	From 24 hours before appearance of first spot until last scab forms (6 days).	No		4
Whooping cough (pertussis)	Bacterium (Bordatella pertussis)	Droplets in the air near infected person.	7–10 days	From 4 days before onset of cough until 3 weeks after.	Yes	Yes	2
German measles (rubella)	Virus (rubella)	Droplets in the air near infected person.	14–21 days (usually 18)	5 days before until 4 days after the appearance of the rash.	Yes	Yes for girls	5
Glandular fever (infectious mononucleosis)	Virus (Epstein– Barr)	Droplets in the air near infected person.	Unknown	Unknown	No		1.3

to be more severe, in adults. However, when a child or adult catches an infection and how severe the attack will be is impossible to forecast. Susceptibility to disease of all kinds is a puzzling and intriguing subject. Some facts are known to be relevant but much remains unexplained. There are racial, familial, and individual variations in susceptibility to infections as well as circumstantial ones. These infectious diseases cause milder illnesses before puberty than after. The closeness of contact and the amount of infected material inhaled or ingested are important. The severity of the disease in the infectious person contacted is not. Sub-clinical, or very mild, disease is as infectious as severe illness. Anyone undernourished, exhausted, or debilitated from some other disease is particularly vulnerable, and emotional well-being and overall standard of living are as important, in this respect, as physical health. It is not clear exactly how these factors operate.

Some of the body's general defence mechanisms are known while others have yet to be identified. The upper respiratory tract is lined by a smooth membrane lubricated by mucus. The cells of the membrane have cilia, which are small, hair-like structures on the surface of the cells. They continually move a thin layer of mucus upward towards the nostrils, trapping and removing inhaled dust, droplets, and particulate matter. Intense cold and cigarette smoke slow down the action of the cilia and it is found that children who live in houses where adults smoke, and the adults themselves, are more likely to develop infections of the respiratory tract. The stomach acid is a powerful defence against swallowed micro-organisms.

Susceptibility to infection varies between individuals and in each individual at different times. The virulence of the infecting micro-organisms also varies from time to time, although it is difficult to be sure how much of this is caused by changes in the organism itself and how much by changes in the overall immunity of the population. A good example of changing virulence is scarlet fever, which used to be a serious and common disease and which is now of no greater importance than the tonsillitis which the same bacterium causes. This is partly owing to the fact that it is sensitive to penicillin and partly owing to improvement in health of the community, but mainly because the bacterium has changed and now causes an altogether milder illness.

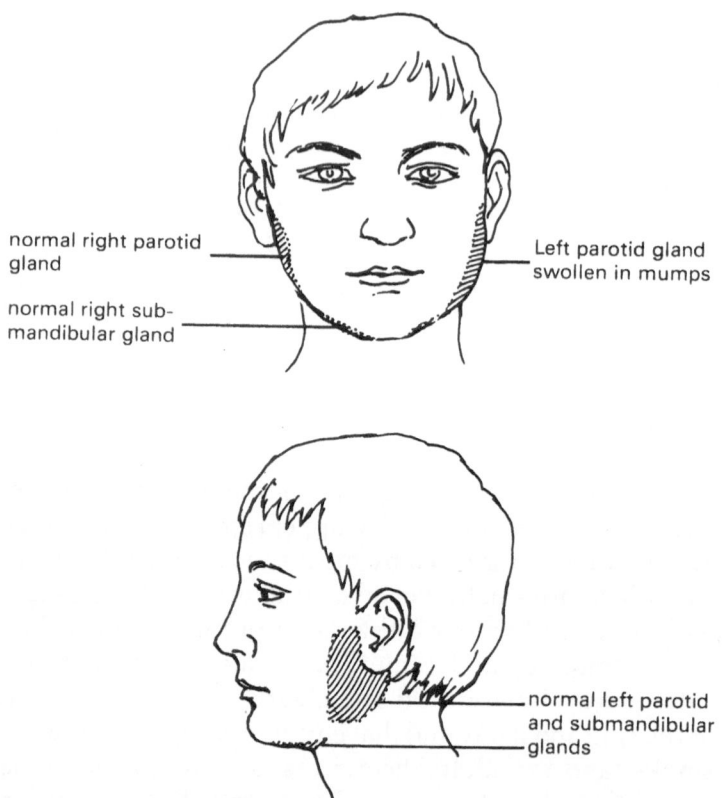

normal right parotid gland

Left parotid gland swollen in mumps

normal right sub-mandibular gland

normal left parotid and submandibular glands

Figure 17.1   The salivary glands

Symptoms

Mumps

Swelling of one or more of the four salivary glands (see Figure 17.1) is usually the first symptom.

They are painful while they are enlarging but once the maximum swelling has been reached the pain lessens. Pain is intensified by the smell or taste of food. The victim develops a fever and general malaise, more intense in adults than children. The whole condition settles in a few days.

Measles

This starts with a fever, cough, and runny nose which may persist for a few days before the main rash appears. This is called the prodromal period. Secondary bacterial infection such as tonsillitis or otitis media may occur during this time. There may also be a rash of whitish spots, known as Koplik's spots, on the inside of the cheeks. During the main illness in addition to fever, cough, and runny nose and eyes there is a bright red, blotchy rash over the whole body. It is most intense over the face and trunk, where it becomes confluent.

A mild attack, or one attenuated by previous immunization, may contain elements of all the symptoms in a greatly diminished form so that it is indistinguishable from a number of other viral illnesses. The rash fades gradually, leaving a faint brownish stain and powdery flaking of the skin. This and all the other symptoms have usually disappeared within ten days.

Chickenpox

The symptoms of chickenpox consist of pink spots, which develop blisters, which then form crusts or scabs. The rash takes two days to develop fully and affects the whole body except the palms and soles of the feet.

Chickenpox is a mild illness in children but adults often have a high fever and feel very miserable for a week or more. The scabs eventually separate and the spots fade, although some may leave permanent, small scars.

Whooping cough

This starts with a slight cough in a well child. The cough develops over a week or ten days, gradually becoming paroxysmal. This means that it occurs in bouts with little or no coughing in between. The paroxysms may be prolonged and severe with retching and a sharp in-drawing of breath at the end of each. In older children this gives rise to the typical 'whoop', which does not occur in babies. Most children vomit during the paroxysms. The cough is often worse at night and is exhausting for both child and parents. The course is very variable. In some, it is so mild that the diagnosis is never considered. An attack may persist for a month or more, with considerable debility.

German measles (rubella)

This is a very mild, insignificant illness in children and even in adults is usually less severe than an attack of flu. It consists of a low-grade fever and faint, pink rash, mainly over the trunk or buttocks. Glands at the back of the neck may be swollen. The rash fades within 36 hours but sometimes adults develop transient swelling and stiffness of the fingers during the subsequent ten days.

Glandular fever

This affects teenagers and causes sore throat, fever and swelling of lymph glands in the neck, under the arms, and in the groins. Occasionally, the liver is affected and transient jaundice develops. It is caused by the EB (Epstein—Barr) virus. The infectivity is not high, and contact with other cases is rarely recalled. The acute phase lasts 2—3 weeks, but in some teenagers a state of weakness and tiredness goes on for months — eventually resolving. There is no specific treatment for glandular fever.

Complications of common infectious diseases

Secondary infections

The commonest complications are bacterial infections of the respiratory tract such as *middle-ear infection* (otitis media) and *acute bronchitis*. They occur in measles and whooping cough and respond well to antibiotics, such as penicillin, but these do not affect the main illness.

Febrile convulsions

These can occur during the course of any febrile illness in a susceptible child (see Chapter 5). They are unusual after the age of 3 years.

Encephalitis

This is a rare inflammatory condition of the brain and its coverings which may follow any viral illness. It is more likely to occur after mumps than the other diseases in this group. The symptoms consist of headache, vomiting, and mild confusion. No treatment other than bed rest is required. It is completely benign and recovery is the rule.

Whooping cough in infants

The danger of whooping cough in very young infants is the very sticky mucus which forms in the air passages and forms plugs. The child attempts to remove these by prolonged paroxysms of coughing during which no air is breathed into the lungs. Brain damage can result from the shortage of oxygen and sometimes fits occur.

The plugs of mucus also may put parts of the lungs out of action because of blocked bronchial tubes — causing infection and pneumonia.

Orchitis in mumps

When the testes are inflamed, the patient is said to be suffering from orchitis. It occurs in some adults with mumps and is an extension of the disease. It is painful and distressing but the patient always recovers and sterility is a very rare sequel indeed, even when the disease has affected both testes. No special treatment is required.

Treatment

There are no drugs available which affect the course of the common infectious diseases under consideration in this section, since they are caused by viruses, which are resistant to antibiotics.

Antibiotics are sometimes used in young children who have been in contact with whooping cough and who have not been immunized, in the hope that complications may be prevented.

Antibiotics are helpful, however, in the treatment of secondary infections such as otitis media and bronchitis.

The treatment of a patient with an infectious disease is therefore directed towards keeping him or her as comfortable as possible while the disease runs its course. Anyone who is feverish will be most comfortable in bed taking copious fluids and occasional aspirin or paracetamol. *Mumps* is usually painful and strongly flavoured food or anything needing chewing is best avoided. *Chickenpox* sometimes itches and calamine lotion is soothing. Hot drinks, steam inhalations, and a steamy atmosphere may help the cough in *whooping cough* and *measles.* There is no particular advantage in keeping someone with measles in the dark unless he or she prefers it.

Infants with whooping cough may need admission to hospital, where oxygen and steam tents are available and the sticky mucus plugs can be removed with a mechanical sucker. Apart from this, patients with infectious diseases are best cared for at home. Many parents are able to recognize *chickenpox* in a child and a physician is not needed. Sometimes *mumps* is equally obvious but it can be confused with swelling of lymph glands in the neck and it is helpful for the diagnosis to be confirmed.

Anyone with a persistent cough, sore throat, or swollen glands should be seen by a doctor so that the diagnosis can be verified, as also should anyone who is severely ill with any of these conditions. Patients suffering from anything but the mildest forms of whooping cough and measles should be seen by a doctor at intervals during the disease to check for complications.

Gastroenteritis

This is the term used for episodes of diarrhoea and vomiting, which appear to be due to infection, even though sometimes no causative organism can be identified.

Viruses are the commonest infecting agents but bacteria are often responsible, as in bacillary dysentery (sonnei group) and food poisoning (salmonella group). Amoebic dysentery is caused by a protozoon.

Gastroenteritis can affect anyone but is commonest in children and travellers. Infants are particularly susceptible because they have no stomach acid to protect them against ingested micro-organisms and because they have no active immunity against the infections. Travellers are meeting organisms which they have not encountered before and to which they have no immunity. The disease is endemic in most communities but does not affect the local adult population.

Gastroenteritis is usually an unpleasant but mild illness which resolves spontaneously. It can be serious in the very young, the very old, or anyone who is debilitated by malnutrition or any other disease. The main danger is dehydration and loss of salt and other electrolytes.

The *symptoms* consist of diarrhoea, vomiting, and abdominal cramps. The stools may be profuse and watery and occasionally contain blood. The abdominal pain is central and colicky, i.e. it comes and goes, and is most obvious just before a bowel action or bout of vomiting.

With rest and frequent clear fluids, a normal healthy individual will recover within 48 hours but may be unable to eat normally for a further three to four days.

In infants, special care is needed to see that fluids are replaced adequately.

The disease is a serious problem in undernourished communities, where it is common because of poor sanitation, hygiene, and contaminated water.

Prevention of gastroenteritis

The general principles of prevention of infectious diseases outlined earlier apply to gastroenteritis, except that immunization is not generally available. Clean water supplies and care in preparation of food are particularly important. Travellers visiting developing countries should not drink local tap water and even bottled and canned drinks cannot always be trusted. All doubtful water should be boiled or sterilized with water purifying tablets. Fruit should be washed.

Breast-fed babies are protected from gastroenteritis partly because the milk is sterile and partly because it contains antibodies against infection.

Stomach acid is an effective defence against ingested micro-organisms and so people should avoid taking antacid medicines unless they are really necessary, especially when travelling.

Anti-infective agents, such as sulphonamides and even antibiotics, have been recommended as prophylactics against infection in travellers. They have been used by sports teams and airline staff and fewer attacks of gastroenteritis result. However, antibiotics alter the natural bacterial flora of the bowel and when the person suffers gastroenteritis it is more severe. They are not recommended for general use. Enterovioform has dangerous side effects and should not be used.

Treatment

Once an attack of gastroenteritis is established, medication of all sorts is best avoided. There are drugs which lessen diarrhoea but they make the patient more ill and in infants can be dangerous. The reason for this is that, in most cases, the infection remains in the bowel and causes little general toxicity. The frequent loose stools sweep the micro-organisms and their irritant toxins away. If the bowel action is slowed, the organisms and their toxins remain in the lumen of the bowel for a longer period and multiply there. They then penetrate the bowel wall, enter the bloodstream, and cause a much more severe, generalized illness. In the same way that cough is useful in removing infected material in bronchitis, diarrhoea benefits the person suffering from gastroenteritis and should not be suppressed.

Bed rest is helpful and it is important to replace the fluids lost. In most people it is enough to take frequent sips of clear fluids: water, fruit juices, or clear soup. If the attack is severe or the patient very young or debilitated, it is necessary to replace salt and other electrolytes as well. It is important not to overdo this. The following solution is suitable:

4 level tablespoons sugar
¾ teaspoon salt
1 teaspoon sodium bicarbonate } accurately measured
1 cup orange juice
Make up to 1 litre (1.76 pints) with boiled water.

If vomiting is severe and prolonged, the patient may need to be admitted to hospital so that fluids can be given intravenously. This is most likely to be necessary in infants under 3 months, who become dangerously dehydrated very rapidly.

Once the diarrhoea and vomiting have stopped, a normal diet may be reintroduced gradually over several days. It is best to avoid milk and strong meats at first and meals should be small.

Most people suffering from gastroenteritis are treated at home and need no medical advice or help.

A physician should be consulted in the following circumstances:

If abdominal pain is severe or persistent and the diagnosis therefore in doubt.

If vomiting predominates and there is severe headache.

If the patient is very young or frail.

If the attack is severe or prolonged.

If the patient has recently returned from abroad.

18
Skin diseases

Skin disorders are an unusual group of diseases. They account for 7% of all consultations in family medicine and considerable attendance at hospital outpatient departments, yet they give rise to little disability, few admissions to hospital, and almost no deaths.

Nearly 75% of consultations are for acute skin infections (boils, cellulitis, impetigo), eczema/dermatitis, and warts, with all other skin diseases being responsible for only a small proportion each.

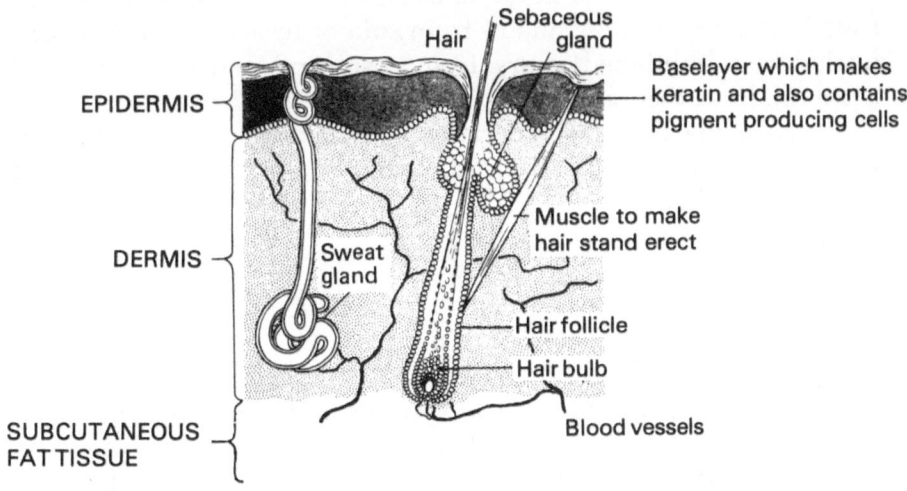

Figure 18.1   The structure of the skin — microscopic section.

The skin consists of two layers called the epidermis and dermis. The epidermis is on the outside and produces a horny material called keratin which forms the outermost protective layer of the body. Friction can initially wear away keratin but then stimulates greater production leading to thicker skin, e.g. on the palms and soles. Special cells in the epidermis produce pigment and are responsible for skin colour. Hair and nails are made of modified keratin (Figure 18.1).

Keratin is kept supple by the secretions of sweat and sebaceous glands. Sweat glands lie deep in the dermis and have ducts which come out on the skin surface. Sweating is an important way of keeping cool. Sebaceous glands lie around and open into hair follicles and produce a greasy substance called sebum. A third type of gland, called the apocrine glands, are situated in the axillae, breasts, and genitals and are concerned with producing characteristic sex smells.

The dermis contains the glands and blood supply for the epidermis. It contains the vital sense receptors which are responsible for receiving information from the outside world about warmth, cold, pain, and pressure, and for the sense of touch which we all rely on.

Causes and effects of disease

With such a large area exposed to the outside world all sorts of external factors can work on the skin and cause disease or injury. Infections from bacteria or viruses, injury from cold or heat or from chemicals (including self-inflicted injury from cosmetics) and other physical agents all have their effects.

Similarly the skin can reflect the external signs of virtually any internal disease. Many rashes, for example, are caused by internal infection or allergy.

Diseases

Acne (See Chapter 6)

This will affect about 80% of adolescents and usually persists from puberty to the late teens or early twenties. In some people, however, it may begin in the thirties and in others it may persist until middle age.

The primary defect is excess keratin production (related to sex hormone concentrations), which blocks the openings of sebaceous glands so letting a blackhead form. These spots occur mainly on the face and centre of the chest and back and can become infected and very inflamed, leading to scarring of the skin in more severe cases.

Measures that will help include sunlight (ultraviolet light peels the skin and so prevents blockage of the sebaceous glands); application of substances like sulphur or retinoic acid (these break up keratin and so help clear blocked sebaceous glands); and the taking of tetracycline drugs for at least six weeks (these destroy the infecting bacteria). Manipulating the diet and washing, or not washing, the skin have no effect.

Allergic rashes

These are common and may occur in one area of the body due to a contact allergy, e.g. from plants, jewellery, or cosmetics or over the whole body from an allergy to some ingested substance (allergen), e.g. foodstuffs, medicines.

The type and extent of the rash varies greatly but from non-plant contact tends to be a local dermatitis, from plant contact a local urticaria (redness and weals as with nettle rash), and from ingested materials a generalized urticaria. In all cases the rash is itchy and will tend to resolve in a few days provided there is no further contact with the allergen.

Contrary to popular belief, for an allergic reaction to take place, a person has to have been in contact with the allergen in the past. Initial contacts give no reaction but make a person sensitive so that future contacts will set off the full allergic reaction.

Once a reaction has taken place antihistamine tablets will help to resolve it and if an allergen has been identified (this is often difficult), then it should be strictly avoided.

Athlete's foot

This is a ringworm-fungus infection of the foot which tends to affect young and middle-aged adult males.

It causes peeling and sogginess of the skin between the outer toes, where it can remain causing only slight irritation. Alternatively it can spread to affect the sole of the foot.

Topical antifungal agents should be used and the area between the toes dried well after bathing. Wearing sandals also helps.

Boils

These are caused by bacterial infection and may occur at any site where there are hair follicles.

A single, isolated boil needs no treatment; it should be left to resolve. Multiple boils may be helped by antibiotics though they usually occur because the infecting germ is harboured in the nose, axillae, or genital area and these areas may need treatment with antibiotic creams or antiseptics.

Multiple boils may rarely be a sign of diabetes.

Impetigo

This is common, especially in children, and is an infection of the outer layer (epidermis) which starts with a purulent blister which soon ruptures, giving a weeping, crusting area. Hands and face are the commonest sites and lesions tend to be golden coloured.

Crusts should be removed by soap and water before applying topical antibiotics three times daily until complete resolution occurs, usually within a few days. Oral antibiotics may need to be taken in the more severe or widespread cases.

Eczema/dermatitis

These are synonymous terms that refer to a special sequence of inflammatory changes which can affect the skin to variable degrees, depending on the site and severity of the disease. Redness, swelling, blisters, weeping, crusting, fissures or splits, scaling, and thickening of the skin may occur, provoking itching and irritation.

In *childhood* constitutional (genetic) factors are thought to be the cause and there is often a family history of asthma or hay fever. About 10% of children are affected to some degree and in most symptoms will be mild and clear up by the age of 5 years. The face, elbow and knee flexures, wrists, and hands are most often affected and it is important to remember that however bad the skin may look all the changes are completely reversible. Treatment with steroid creams is usually given and they act to suppress the inflammatory process that is taking place in the skin. Although these creams will clear the skin they will not cure it (only time will), and also if used to excess for long periods they can actually damage the skin themselves, apart from causing other problems like stunting a child's growth.

In *adults* eczema may be due to specific external factors affecting the skin and can either be a true allergic reaction to a chemical or other substance or a reaction to an irritant, e.g. washing up powders or liquids, that is damaging the skin directly. In these cases topical steroid creams will help but unless the irritant or allergy producing substance is identified and then strictly avoided the eczema will continually recur.

Psoriasis

This affects about 2% of people at some time in their lives. The exact cause is not known, although it is thought to be an inherited disorder.

The first attack usually occurs in the late teens or the twenties and then the disease runs a lifelong relapsing and remitting course.

Typically there are numerous areas of skin which consist of sharply demarcated, raised, red, silver-scaled circular plaques. Knees, elbows, and scalp are common sites but the whole body can be affected when the disease is particularly active. Nails often become thickened and pitted and in about one in twenty sufferers arthritis will develop.

Psoriasis is not infectious and is not a sign of internal disease. In most people it can be helped by treatment (though there is no permanent cure) and in many it can disappear as mysteriously as it arose. When it does clear the skin is left unblemished.

Natural sunlight often helps and special ultraviolet ray therapy is also beneficial. There are no other general measures that will make much difference. Tar preparations applied daily, though messy, are effective, as is dithranol applied to chronic plaques of the limbs and trunk. Steroid creams are also very useful but if used excessively can damage the skin and when stopped will often be followed by relapse.

Warts

These are an infectious viral disease that affect about 10% of the population at any one time. They virtually all eventually disappear by themselves. In children the large majority disappear in about 6 months, while in adults about 2—3 years is the outside limit. The disappearance is caused by the virus itself getting old and dying and also by the body developing immunity and destroying it. If warts are removed by treatment before immunity has developed then the person is very likely to catch more.

Verrucae are warts on the feet and, unlike other warts, they may become painful as they are pressed into the skin of the soles by the pressure of walking.

There is no drug effective against the wart virus and in most cases treatments have poorer results than if the wart is left alone. Left alone the wart is generally painless and will resolve without leaving any scars. Treatment may well be painful and may leave a scar. Unless a wart is producing pain or deformity treatment is best avoided.

As so many people have warts spread within the population cannot be prevented. Wearing a waterproof plaster or plastic shoe to cover a verruca allows children to continue swimming without being too great a source of virus for other swimmers to catch.

Risks and action

Keep your skin clean but beware of overuse of soaps which can remove the body's natural skin fats.

Avoid excessive use of cosmetics/perfumes/bubble baths, etc., especially if you have a history of allergy or skin disease.

Judicious exposure to sunlight helps the body produce vitamin D and may improve acne or psoriasis. Prolonged over-exposure may produce skin cancer and may worsen psoriasis.

19

Endocrine disorders

These are the results of malfunctioning of those glands in the body which produce hormones. *Hormones* are chemical substances which are present in tiny amounts in the body but which have the important function of controlling the rate and nature of many of the complex processes which are necessary for life. Glands may produce either too much hormone, as in the case of *hyperthyroidism*, or too little hormone, as in the case of severe *diabetes*, when the body produces little or no insulin.

Endocrine disorders, particularly those arising from a shortage of the particular hormone, are some of the most rewarding conditions for a physician to treat since it is possible to replace the missing substance quite easily and return a seriously ill person to normal health. However, it is necessary to continue supervision for the rest of that person's life to be sure that the correct amount of hormone is being administered continuously.

Apart from diabetes and thyroid disorders, the other endocrine disorders are rare and the average family physician can expect to see only one or two cases in an entire professional lifetime. Unfortunately, there is little evidence that *obesity* is an endocrine disorder, and although it would be good to treat fat persons with an effective pill, it is certainly not yet amenable to hormone treatment.

Diabetes

What is it?

In diabetes there is too much glucose (sugar) in the blood because the body is unable to deal with (metabolize) the glucose. This results in the excess blood sugar 'spilling over' into the urine, where it may be easily detected by simple tests.

There are broadly two types of diabetes. The *juvenile-onset type* found in children and young adults (under 40 years) is an acute illness and needs diet and insulin treatment. The *mature-onset type* in people over 40 years of age, often with little or no symptoms, can be managed by diet, with or without drugs taken by mouth. The distinction between these two types is not complete: some young people can be managed without insulin whilst some elderly patients will require insulin treatment at some stage of the condition.

Who gets it?

Diabetes is common in affluent Western countries. The 'juvenile-onset' type makes up only 10—20% of the total. The 'mature-onset' type is the more usual form and increases steadily with age, so that while one person in every 2000 in the 40—49 year age group will develop the condition each year, in the 70—80 year age group two in every 1000 will be newly affected each year. This means that a family physician in the UK or USA will diagnose 3—6 new patients and look after up to 60 diabetic patients each year in his or her practice.

There is a family tendency to diabetes and anyone who has a close relative with diabetes is at extra risk. Most 'maturity-onset' diabetics are overweight and this is a reason for the high rate of diabetes in our overfed community. Certain drugs may also exacerbate a diabetic tendency and any woman who has given birth to a very large baby i.e. over 4.5 kg (10 lbs) is at risk.

What is its importance?

It is important to diagnose diabetes and to treat the condition as carefully as possible because patients suffering from diabetes are liable to a range of complications. The reasons are not clear but other factors in addition to the blood sugar concentration are involved. Since more people are living into old age and obesity is so widespread the rate of diabetes will continue to rise and more will be at risk of developing complications.

What are its features?

The two types of diabetes usually present in different ways.

The *child or young adult* commonly develops an acute illness with increasing thirst, passing large quantities of urine and losing weight through fluid loss. He or she may become rapidly worse, with vomiting and abdominal pain, and may lapse into unconsciousness. This is a medical emergency which requires urgent hospital admission for rehydration and insulin treatment. Left untreated the patient would die within a short while.

The *older person* may have no symptoms at all and the condition may be diagnosed only by routine urine testing. Alternatively, they may develop thirst and pass excessive quantities of urine as outlined above but be less seriously ill, or they may present with some complication.

Because diabetes lowers resistence to infection this may take the form of soreness and itching in the genital areas due to a thrush infection, multiple boils, or even tuberculosis of the lungs. Alternatively, the condition may present with cramp in the limbs, weakness and heaviness of the legs, pins and needles, an ulcerated foot, impotence in men, impairment of vision or just a general feeling of malaise due to the effects of the diabetes on the nervous system and the circulatory system. The physician will wish to test a urine sample for sugar whenever there is even a remote possibility of diabetes causing the symptoms.

The diagnosis will be confirmed by measuring the blood sugar concentration, which gives a better indication of the severity of the disease, and the physician will check for any signs of complications.

What happens?

Diabetes can be controlled but not cured. There is no known cure for diabetes. It will persist for life even though in mild forms it may be completely controlled by diet alone. It is usually relatively easy to remove the symptoms and improve well-being but it may be difficult to control the blood sugar levels completely.

The diabetic is at an increased risk of developing complications such as coronary heart disease; blockage of arteries in the legs, leading to poor circulation and even gangrene; cataract (dullness of the lens of the eye) and damage to the retina (nerve layer) of the eye which lead to impairment of vision; damage to the nervous system, causing problems in feeling and mobility; weakness of the kidneys; and increased susceptibility to infections of all kinds. The rates of most of these complications are reduced by good control of the diabetic condition.

What to do

Prevention is limited. Apart from choosing the right parents and dying early the chief hope is to avoid becoming obese. Most maturity-onset diabetics are considerably overweight and diabetes in many can be controlled when their ideal weight target is achieved.

Recent onset of thirst, passing more urine, tiredness, itching in genital areas, and possible weight loss are signals for an early medical consultation and a urine test for sugar levels.

Who does what?

If the diagnosis of diabetes is established then it is important that the family, especially the cook of the household, becomes familiar with the dietary requirements of the patient. There are many types of *diabetic diet* but essentially they are all concerned with restricting the total calorie intake and especially the intake of carbohydrates such as in sugar, cakes, sweets, and pastries. Fat should be restricted to reduce possible complications in the heart and blood vessels. *Smoking* must be strongly discouraged in diabetics because of the increased risks of these complications. *Care of the feet*, including regular visits to the chiropodist, helps to prevent troubles such as ulcers.

Diabetics should *test their urine regularly for sugar* as advised and keep a record of the results. These tests are easily and quickly done (without any mess) with tablets or testing strips.

Those needing *insulin* will be instructed on care of the syringe and needles and the techniques of injection. A diabetic will need to know what type of insulin and dose of insulin he or she must take, depending on the medical advice and his or her own personal requirements in special circumstances such as on taking extra exercise. He or she will also need to know how it feels when the blood sugar level drops too low, as may occur with insulin. This situation is known as a 'hypo' (hypoglycaemia) and it is important that the diabetic and family recognize what is happening so that the diabetic can take some extra sugar or chocolate to raise the low blood sugar. If this is not done confusion and loss of consciousness may develop, needing intravenous sugar given in hospital. Some diabetics now carry test strips which respond to a drop of blood and change colour according to the blood sugar level. This may be measured by a small electronic gadget and permits a closer control of blood sugar.

Maturity-onset diabetics may need tablets in addition to a strict diet and they need to know how many tablets to take each day and also be aware of the possible risk of a 'hypo'. These drugs, which increase metabolism of sugar, may have other side effects such as nausea, giddiness, and an unfortunate tendency for the face to flush if alcohol is taken. Perhaps this is just as well since alcoholic drinks in any significant quantity are likely to upset the dietary control.

If a diabetic becomes ill for any other reason, especially if the illness includes vomiting and loss of the ability to take food and fluids, then a physician should be consulted. Insulin dosage may need to be increased and it is *important not to omit an insulin injection* in the mistaken belief that it will not be required because the patient is not eating or drinking. Frequent, small amounts of glucose in water will often be acceptable when the patient is unable to retain food.

Diabetics should attend a physician regularly to check progress. How often will depend on circumstances and may vary from every month to only once or twice a year. This supervision may be carried out by the family physician alone or in co-operation with a consultant.

The most important person in the management of diabetes is the diabetic. If he or she takes the trouble to learn about the disease, understand its effects, stick to the appropriate dietary measures, take the prescribed drugs, stop smoking, take some regular exercise, and look after his or her feet and general health, then he or she is likely to do well and avoid or delay the onset of complications. No physician, nurse, or clinic can manage diabetics satisfactorily without active co-operation from the diabetic.

Thyroid disorders

What are they?

The thyroid gland produces a hormone, thyroxine, which controls the rates at which the body burns up food and at which other biochemical processes occur. An *overactive gland* acts as an accelerator and an *underactive gland* acts as a brake. The effects which disorders of the thyroid gland have on the body may be readily understood in these terms.

Hypothyroidism (myxoedema) [underactive thyroid gland]

This condition is caused by a deficiency of the thyroid hormone. In most cases this occurs for no obvious reason but, on occasion, it may follow treatment of hyperthyroidism, if the thyroid has been destroyed by surgery or radio-iodine treatment. Women are affected ten times as often as men and it is uncommon under the age of 45 years. A family physician may expect to see five to ten patients with this condition at any one time.

What are its features?

Hypothyroidism is an insidious condition because the gland fails slowly and the effects may be inconspicuous. It may be very difficult to diagnose, especially if the physician is being seen often for other reasons and if he or she fails to appreciate the very gradual changes which occur. These include increasing weight, dryness and loss of the hair, a hoarse voice, coarsening of the skin, and bagginess around the eyes. There may be tiredness and weakness, aches and pains, dislike of cold weather, constipation and failing memory. Unfortunately these are all normal symptoms commonly experienced by many, especially if they are elderly.

What happens?

Once the condition has been suspected a blood test will confirm the diagnosis. Without treatment the patient will gradually get worse and be at increasing risk of heart disease and of hypothermia in winter. *Hypothermia* is a condition in which the patient is unable to maintain his or her normal body temperature and it may be fatal.

With treatment — thyroxine tablets by mouth for life — the outlook is excellent and the condition can be completely controlled.

Hyperthyroidism (overactive thyroid gland)

This condition is caused by an excess of thyroid hormone. It is not as simple a condition to understand as hypothyroidism since the mechanism whereby the gland becomes overactive is more complex. Women are affected five times as often as men. One group of patients may be affected in early adult life, whilst others are not affected until old age. It is less common than hypothyroidism.

What are its features?

Younger persons tend to present with severe weight loss, increasing nervousness, protruding eyes, swelling of the thyroid gland (goitre), a dislike of hot weather, and irregular or absent periods in women. A severe emotional upset appears to precipitate the disease occasionally and it may be difficult to differentiate from an anxiety state in some patients since they may also develop palpitations, sweats, diarrhoea, and a tremor; all of which may be produced by anxiety alone. Diagnosis is confirmed by a blood test.

The diagnosis may be more difficult in *elderly* persons who often do not show the typical features of the disease and may present with unexplained heart failure, irregularity of the pulse, or even mental disturbances.

What happens?

Although some mild cases will recover within a few months on their own and may never be diagnosed, most patients will require treatment.

Carbimazole will suppress the overactive thyroid gland and may tide the patient over for a year or two until the disease 'burns itself out'.

However, if drug treatment fails in the younger person, if there is a large thyroid swelling causing discomfort, or if the person is unwilling to take drugs for a long period then an operation to remove most of the thyroid gland, *thyroidectomy*, is very effective.

In patients over 45, i.e. beyond the reproductive age, the most elegant treatment is a simple drink of water containing the tasteless, odourless substance, *radioactive iodine*. This is selectively taken up by the thyroid gland and gradually destroys it. It works rather slowly and it is difficult to calculate the precise dose required, so the patient has to be followed up carefully. Sometimes a further dose is required.

It may be that after removal or destruction of the thyroid gland, a state of hypothyroidism develops years later. This will need control by thyroxine tablets.

20

Cystitis and gynaecological disorders

The genitourinary tract comprises the kidneys, ureters, bladder, urethra, and all the sex organs. These are shown in Figures 20.1 and 20.2 and in Chapter 2.

The most common diseases affecting these organs are infections:

Cystitis — infection of the bladder.
Pyelitis — infection of the ureters.
Salpingitis — infection of the Fallopian tubes.
Vaginitis — infection of the vagina.
Urethritis — infection of the urethra.
Prostatitis — infection of the prostate gland.
Epididymitis — infection of the epididymis.

The word *nephritis* is used to describe certain diseases of the kidney which are not due to infection.

Renal and ureteric calculi (*stones*) are common and so are benign tumours of the uterus (*fibroids*), and enlargement of the prostate gland.

The more serious conditions *renal failure* and *cancers* are rare.

Infections of the bladder and ureters (cystitis and pyelitis)

These are caused by bacteria. They are most common in sexually active adult women and in them the bacteria enter from the outside along the urethra. Bacteria can also be carried to the urinary tract in

257

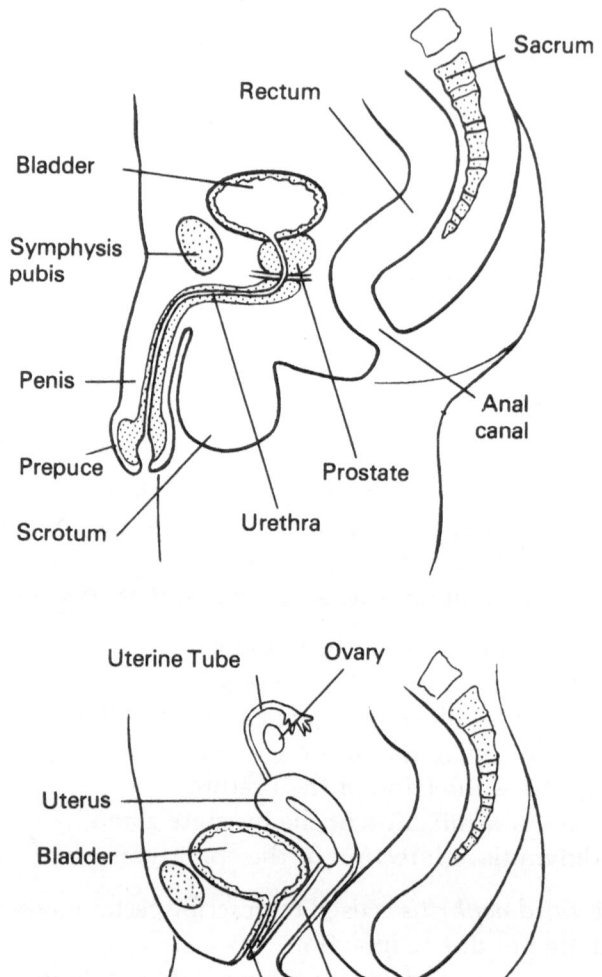

(a)

(b)

Figure 20.1   The genital tract. (a) Male; (b) female.

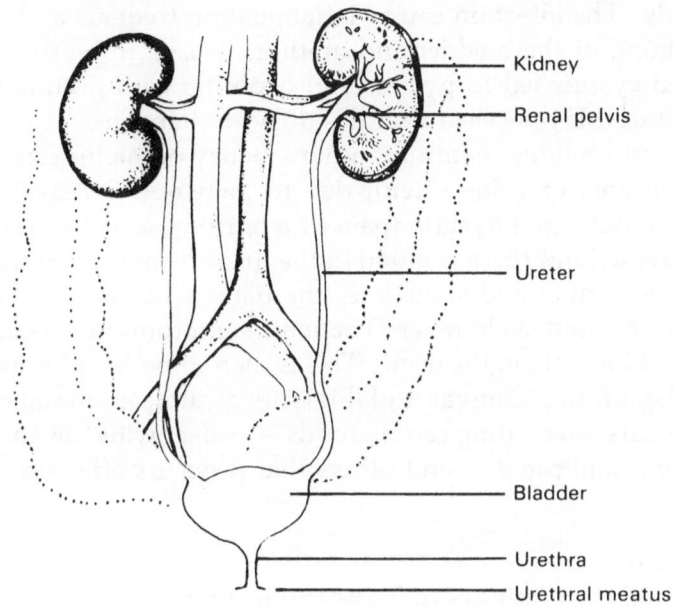

Figure 20.2 The urinary tract.

the bloodstream and this is the usual route in infants and men. In infants and the elderly, infections of the urinary tract are slightly more common in males; but between 3 months and 65 years they are far more common in females. The incidence is highest in women aged between 15 and 40, with a peak in the early twenties.

Occasional attacks of cystitis in adult women are so common as to be part of normal life and have no sinister significance. They are unpleasant and may cause the sufferer much misery but they are never life threatening and have no serious long-term effects.

Repeated urinary infections, especially in a child, may be an indication of a structural abnormality in the urinary tract and further investigation is needed. This usually includes an X-ray (intravenous pyelogram, IVP) or cystoscopy (see p. 262).

Cystitis

Although the bladder and ureters are all part of a single system, cystitis usually occurs without obvious pyelitis and is therefore considered separately. The infection causes inflammation (redness and swelling) of the lining of the bladder and urethra. It used to be thought that neglected cystitis led to pyelitis and nephritis with eventual kidney damage but it is now clear that this does not happen.

The most obvious *symptoms* are frequency of micturition (passing small amounts of urine often), due to increased irritability of the bladder muscle, and dysuria (pain or a burning sensation on passing urine). Sometimes there is blood in the urine from the raw surface of the bladder lining and sometimes the patient has lower abdominal pain, nausea, and slight fever. The same symptoms may occur in the absence of bacteria in the urine. This is then sometimes known as the *urethral syndrome*. The cause of this is not at all clear but some women find it occurs after eating certain foods — coffee, wine, and acid fruits have been implicated — and others that it occurs after sexual intercourse.

What to do

Cystitis and the urethral syndrome can be prevented if there is a precipitating cause and if that cause can be identified and avoided. This is not always easy but if the symptom seems closely to follow sexual activity, it may be possible to use lubricants and alter the technique of intercourse so that the urethra does not get bruised during love-making. A high fluid intake, emptying the bladder after intercourse and a high standard of hygiene may all help.

The symptoms of cystitis may be relieved by bed rest, warmth (e.g. a hot water bottle), plentiful fluids, and analgesics such as paracetamol or aspirin. It is also helpful to render the urine alkaline by taking sodium bicarbonate (one teaspoonful in a cup of water) or potassium citrate mixture.

If the symptoms persist or are severe or recurrent, medical advice should be sought.

Untreated cystitis in adult women resolves without treatment in time but the symptoms may be prolonged and most physicians prescribe a course of antibiotics.

Pyelitis and pyelonephritis

Bacterial infection affects the ureters and renal pelvis on one or both sides. It is most likely to occur in pregnant women and in anyone with a structural abnormality in the urinary tract, although it can affect anyone. It is a much more serious condition than cystitis and if neglected can lead to kidney damage. Tuberculosis used to be a common cause but is now rare in developed countries.

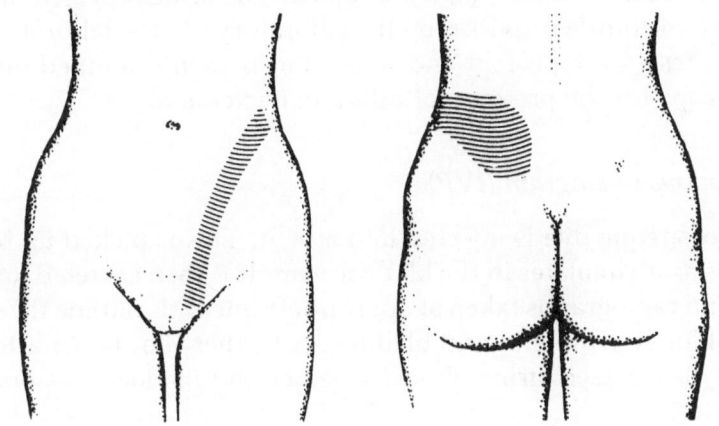

Figure 20.3   Site of pain (shaded area) in pyelitis and kidney stone.

Symptoms
Acute pyelitis causes a high fever with attacks of shaking (rigors) and abdominal and loin pain. This corresponds with the position of the affected organs (see Figure 20.3). The severity of the illness is due to the presence of bacteria in the bloodstream. If it is not efficiently treated, the drainage system of the kidney (the renal pelvis and ureter) can become distended and distorted, predisposing the patient to further attacks of pyelitis. The kidney tissue may also be damaged, leading to hypertension (high blood pressure) and eventually to renal failure.

What to do
Prevention — The incidence of pyelitis in pregnancy has been greatly reduced by the routine examination of the urine for bacteria in early pregnancy. Apart from this it is not possible to forecast who is likely to develop pyelitis and it cannot therefore be prevented.

   Treatment — This is directed at eradicating the bacteria with antibiotics and making sure that the urinary tract is structurally normal. Recurrent attacks can sometimes be prevented by the use of antibiotics for a prolonged period.

Investigation of the urinary tract

Examination of the urine

A midstream or 'clean-catch' specimen is needed so that contamination from mucus around the vulva is avoided. The urine is passed directly into a sterile bottle provided by the laboratory. At the laboratory the urine is tested for protein and sugar and is then examined under a microscope for the presence of cells and bacteria.

Intravenous pyelogram (IVP)

A radio-opaque dye is injected into a vein. This is picked up by the kidneys as it circulates in the bloodstream. It is then excreted into the urine and radiographs taken at appropriate intervals outline the shape of the kidneys, ureters, and bladder. A further film taken after the patient has passed urine shows whether the bladder has emptied completely.

Cystoscopy

This is usually performed under a general anaesthetic by a surgeon using a fine periscope-like tube, which is passed along the urethra. It allows him to examine the lining of the bladder and the openings of the ureters. He can remove small pieces of tissue (biopsy samples) for examination in the laboratory. If there are warts, or papillomata, in the bladder they can be destroyed through the cystoscope by diathermy. He can also pass a fine tube up one or both ureters to obtain separate samples of urine from each kidney or to inject radio-opaque dye so that radiographs can be taken showing the outline of the ureters and kidneys.

Blood tests

The state of the kidneys is reflected in the level of waste products, especially urea, in the blood. If the kidneys are damaged and failing to excrete the waste products efficiently, the level of urea in the blood rises (uraemia). This has a depressing effect on bone marrow and such patients are usually also anaemic.

Vaginitis and vulvitis (inflammation of vagina and vulva)

The healthy vulva and vagina normally contain a mixture of micro-organisms, which form a balanced community living in symbiosis with their human host. They cause no symptoms and in this situation can be said to be non-pathogenic, i.e. causing no disease. This is in contrast to the renal tract (kidneys, ureters, and bladder) which is sterile and should contain no organisms. The status quo in the vagina is dependent on the hormonal state of the woman, which is responsible for the quality of the mucosal lining, the mucus which it produces, and its resultant acidity. The situation changes at different ages and at different stages in the menstrual cycle. It can also be altered by trauma and by chemicals, like bath salts. It is important to remember these basic principles as vaginitis often develops more as a result of changes in the vagina itself, rendering it more susceptible, than to the arrival of an overwhelming number of pathogenic (disease-producing) organisms.

This increased susceptibility is particularly seen in the sexually active young woman. Inexperience and a youthful partner often mean that intercourse takes place before she is fully aroused and the vulva and vagina appropriately lubricated and swollen. This means that the thrusting penis has an abrasive effect on the vulva and vagina, making them sore and bruising the urethral meatus, possibly contributing to the *urethral syndrome*. This soreness alters the mucosal lining and the mucus production changes so that normally non-pathogenic organisms may multiply and cause symptoms. Pregnant women, women taking oral contraceptives, and diabetics are more susceptible to *vaginal thrush* (infection with the yeast *Candida albicans*), possibly because of changes in acidity and sugar content of the mucus.

Elderly women, in whom hormonal changes have led to a thinning (atrophy) of the tissues and lessening of lubrication, are particularly subject to vaginitis. Soap, bath salts, douches, and deodorants may all interfere with the natural resistance of these tissues to infection. *Vaginal thrush* often develops after a course of antibiotics taken for a quite different condition. It appears likely that the antibiotics upset the balance of nature in the vagina by destroying some of the natural inhabitants, allowing others to flourish.

Some vaginal infections develop in a healthy vagina because the micro-organism is overpowering. This is particularly true of the venereal diseases, especially *gonorrhoea*, and of *trichomonas vaginalis infection*, which is sometimes transmitted by sexual intercourse and sometimes by other means, such as infected towels. Once one of these infections is established in the vagina, the normal balanced ecology and resistance to infection is destroyed and other organisms flourish so that it is sometimes impossible to say which is causing the symptoms.

The importance of vaginitis lies mainly in the misery it causes. Except in gonorrhoea, there are no serious long-term effects.

What are its features?

The *symptoms* consist of soreness, itching, and discharge which vary according to the causative agent. The discharge must be distinguished from the normal production of mucus which varies with age, menstrual cycle, sexual activity, and a number of other factors. Every woman learns to recognize what is normal for her. Children often produce vaginal mucus from an early age. Provided it is not profuse, thick and yellow (like pus), blood stained, or associated with soreness, it should be left alone.

In thrush, irritation predominates and the discharge is white and curdy. In trichomonas the discharge is thick and yellow or greenish and there is more soreness and less irritation. In gonorrhoea, the discharge may be profuse, thin, and yellow and associated with dysuria and lower abdominal pain. Often there is no discharge at all. Commonly, vaginitis is associated with infection with a mixture of organisms and the symptoms are variable.

What to do

Prevention

It is sensible for any woman to avoid things which she knows cause vaginal soreness. These may include bubble baths, nylon pants, and rubber contraceptives, if she is allergic to rubber. These factors will be different for each individual. The frequency of vaginal thrush after antibiotics is another good reason for not taking them unless they are really necessary. A new look at their sexual technique may enable a couple to prevent further vaginitis in the woman. In certain infections, especially venereal diseases and trichomonas, it is important to treat the male partner at the same time as treating the woman if reinfection later is to be avoided. Any other partners must, of course, also be treated.

Treatment
It is sometimes only necessary to avoid further irritants such as soap or sex for a while for the condition to resolve spontaneously. A table-spoonful of salt or vinegar in the bath water is helpful. If these fail, medical help will be needed.

Further investigations such as swabs and smears may be needed to elucidate the diagnosis, but if the symptoms sound as though the cause is thrush then many physicians will prescribe a course of antifungal pessaries in the first instance and only proceed to further investigations if the condition fails to respond. The treatment then will depend on the identification of the cause of the problem. Infection can be treated with creams or pessaries used locally in the vagina or in some cases with tablets taken by mouth. The acidity of the vagina can be increased by lactic acid pessaries which hasten a return to normal. Oestrogen creams may be helpful for senile, or atrophic, vaginitis. If the symptoms are persistent or recurrent, then further investigation may be needed.

If veneral disease is suspected or diagnosed, special swabs and blood tests are necessary and have to be repeated after treatment. Often more than one of these infections, such as gonorrhoea and syphilis, are present at the same time and both must be fully treated if serious sequelae are to be avoided. It is also extremely important for all possible contacts to be traced and checked for infection.

Salpingitis

This is a bacterial infection of the Fallopian tubes. It is relatively uncommon, affecting less than one woman in every 1000 each year. A variety of different bacteria may be responsible. Tuberculosis used to be a common cause but now that the overall incidence of the disease has declined, it has become rare. Almost any pathogenic bacterium (one causing disease in humans) can cause salpingitis, reaching the site by way of the vagina and uterus or the bloodstream. It is slightly more likely to occur in a woman with an intrauterine contraceptive device than in one without. Gonorrhoea is the only venereal disease to cause salpingitis.

Apart from the acute illness, the main importance of salpingitis is that in some women it causes the tubes to become blocked by scar tissue and the woman may be unable to conceive.

What are the features?

The symptoms are: lower abdominal pain, vaginal discharge, and deep dyspareunia (pain with sexual intercourse). The woman may be acutely ill with a fever and nausea or vomiting.

What to do

In the early stages, salpingitis can be treated successfully with antibiotics but occasionally pus collects, forming an abscess in the Fallopian tube and this may have to be drained by an open operation.

Male infections

Urethritis

This occurs in men and women and is usually due to a venereal infection; NSU (non-specific urethritis) or gonorrhoea. It is best investigated and treated at a special clinic because of the possibility of other coexisting disease, especially syphilis.

Epididymitis

This is sometimes associated with venereal infection but may also be caused by other micro-organisms. It causes painful swelling in the scrotum and responds to treatment with antibiotics. Tuberculosis used to be a common cause but is now rare.

Orchitis

This is an inflammation of the testes and is most commonly caused by the mumps virus. There is no treatment and although it is painful, it always resolves spontaneously.

The uterus (womb)

The commonest problems affecting the uterus are not diseases but disorders of function. A uterus and all the related organs — ovaries, Fallopian tubes, and vagina — may be structurally normal and healthy but still give rise to incapacitating pain or bleeding which is heavy and erratic.

The menstrual cycle is very variable and individual. It is not normal for a healthy adult woman to have no menstrual loss at all, nor to bleed continuously, but between these extremes almost any pattern is compatible with health.

With modern drugs and surgical techniques it should not be necessary for a woman to suffer intolerably from pain or bleeding but what is intolerable varies from one woman to another. Most doctors feel that no woman should be allowed to bleed so much that she becomes anaemic or suffer so much pain and bleeding that her normal life is disrupted.

Dysmenorrhoea (painful periods)

This consists of cramp-like, lower abdominal pain, sometimes accompanied by backache, usually occurring on the first day of menstruation. It is most common in young women, starting some months or a year after the onset of menstruation. It is not known what causes it. It is said to be an indication that ovulation is taking place but is not a reliable sign. It causes the greatest problems in those who are under emotional stress and it is important to include an examination of this aspect of a girl's life if her dysmenorrhoea is to be relieved. Dysmenorrhoea is not caused by physical disease but if a woman is worried about whether she is normal, it may be helpful for a physician to examine her so that she can be reassured.

Fatigue and constipation are sometimes contributory causes.

What to do
Treatment. Simple analgesics (pain relievers) are effective if taken early enough, before the pain becomes severe, in adequate dosage and repeated regularly. Paracetamol every 4 hours or aspirin every 4 hours are appropriate. If the onset of the pain can be forecast, the first dose should be taken an hour or more before. Codeine should be avoided

because it may cause constipation. If these measures fail, a physician may prescribe alternative analgesics or hormone tablets, either an oral contraceptive or non-contraceptive hormone, to be taken in a cyclical way to fit in with menstruation. Sometimes the problem may not be severe enough to justify continuous hormone treatment. It can then be used for a few weeks or months at a time to cover important events such as holidays or exams.

Dysmenorrhoea is less common in women of over 25 but it does occur and there is no truth in the saying that it always goes once a woman has had a baby.

Menorrhagia

This is the term used to describe heavy menstrual bleeding. There is no precise definition of what constitutes menorrhagia and one woman may consider normal what another finds excessive. In the absence of other symptoms such as bleeding between the periods (intermenstrual bleeding) or vaginal discharge, it is rarely associated with disease. However, it is advisable for every woman to have a vaginal examination and cervical smear before embarking on hormone treatment for menorrhagia.

What to do
If she does not wish to take hormones, or if there is a medical reason why she should not, then she should at least have a blood test occasionally to check whether she is anaemic and take iron tablets if necessary.

If menorrhagia is severe and hormones are contraindicated or fail to control it, a hysterectomy may be the only choice to putting up with it. It is usual for a D and C (dilatation and curettage) to be done first. This consists of stretching the cervix and scraping out the lining of the uterus with a spoon-like instrument (curette) for examination in the laboratory. Occasionally this procedure itself relieves the menorrhagia, at least for a time.

Diseases of the uterus (womb)

The commonest diseases are cervical erosions and polyps, the rarest are cancer of the cervix and body of the uterus. The following symptoms may indicate disease and should not be ignored:

Bleeding between periods.
Bleeding after intercourse.
Abnormal vaginal discharge.
Unusually prolonged menstrual loss.

Cervical erosion

In this condition, the surface cells of the mucosa covering the cervix are deficient and the cervix appears red and granular instead of pink and smooth and shiny. It looks a bit like a superficial graze on a child's knee. In some women this condition is present from birth (congenital erosion) and is of no importance. In others, it develops after pregnancy or infection and is associated with intermenstrual or post-coital bleeding (bleeding between periods or after intercourse) and with vaginal discharge. It may heal spontaneously when the infection is treated but if it persists, cautery may be necessary. In this, the surface cells are burnt away and healing encouraged.

The contraceptive pill does not cause a cervical erosion but if one develops in a woman taking the pill, healing may be delayed until she stops taking it for a few months.

Cervical polyps

These are small, benign tumours which may cause irregular bleeding and should be removed. This is usually a simple matter and can be done without an anaesthetic in an outpatient clinic or while carrying out a D and C.

Fibroids

These are benign, solid tumours of the uterus which cause it to enlarge and may be associated with menorrhagia. Usually they cause no symptoms and can be safely left alone but sometimes their sheer size causes symptoms of a swollen abdomen or pressure on the bladder and then they are best removed by hysterectomy.

Cancer of the cervix

This is a slowly growing cancer which develops in the cells on the surface of the cervix. It is not at all common and if diagnosed at an early stage can be cured. It affects women aged between 35 and 50 but changes in the cells of the cervix can sometimes be detected a long time before they become truly malignant. The symptoms are similar to those of a cervical erosion: intermenstrual or post-coital bleeding and sometimes increased vaginal discharge. Anyone with these symptoms should see a doctor, although they are much more likely to be caused by the common erosion than by the rare cancer.

Prevention consists of taking cervical smears at intervals from the age of about 20 years. This enables abnormal cells to be identified at a premalignant stage, when they can easily be removed. Treatment of the cancer itself is by hysterectomy, radiotherapy, or both.

Cancer of the body of the uterus is even more rare than that of the cervix. It occurs in women after the menopause and shows itself by post-menopausal bleeding, which should always be investigated, although it is most likely to be due to a benign cause such as senile vaginitis. Treatment is similar to that for cancer of the cervix.

Hysterectomy

The surgical removal of the uterus; this is the standard treatment for intractable and disabling menorrhagia and for cancer of the uterine cervix and body. With modern techniques it has become a simple and safe operation and is undertaken increasingly.

When the operation is performed for a benign condition, then it is usual to leave the ovaries so that the woman's hormonal state is unaffected. If it is performed for the treatment of cancer, or if there are practical difficulties, e.g. due to scar tissue in the pelvis from previous infection or surgery, then it may be necessary for the ovaries to be removed as well. The operation is usually carried out through an incision in the lower abdomen. If there is an associated prolapse with weakness of the pelvic muscles, and a repair operation is planned to correct this then the whole operation may be carried out through the vagina: vaginal hysterectomy, and there is no abdominal incision. The cervix is removed with the rest of the uterus and the vagina stitched over to form a blind end.

If the ovaries are retained, the woman experiences little or no constitutional disturbance after the operation once the wound has healed. Normal physical and sexual activities can be resumed within two to four weeks. Fatigue and emotional disturbance are no greater than for any other operation unless the woman was under stress already. If the operation is carried out for menorrhagia and the menorrhagia was associated with emotional disturbance then the operation will cure only the menorrhagia. The emotional disturbance may continue and then be attributed to the operation itself. It has been found that depression after hysterectomy is more likely to occur when the uterus that is removed is structurally normal than when it is diseased, e.g. by cancer.

If the ovaries are removed in a pre-menopausal woman, she may experience a sudden menopause with violent hot flushes and transient reduction in libido. This does not occur if the ovaries are retained. In fact, libido may increase once the risk of pregnancy is removed.

The prostate gland

This is shaped like a doughnut and lies at the base of the bladder around the urethra, which passes through the middle of it. Behind it is the rectum and in front, the pubic bone. The ducts from the seminal vesicles pass through it from behind (see Figure 20.1(a)). It produces a small amount of fluid which is added to the semen during ejaculation.

Infection of the prostate gland (prostatitis)

This can be caused by micro-organisms, which reach it along the urethra or in the bloodstream. It can be caused by NSU or gonorrhoea. It is treated with antibiotics. In NSU prolonged or repeated courses of treatment may be necessary.

Benign enlargement of the prostate

This occurs to some extent in every man over 40 but only one in ten develops symptoms from it and then not usually until 60 years of age or over. The symptoms are due to obstruction to the outflow of urine from the bladder.

What are the features?
A man with an enlarged prostate will:

Have a poor stream when passing urine.

Take a long time to pass urine, often having to wait for the flow to start.

Need to pass urine more often.

Find that he can often pass more urine a few minutes after apparently emptying his bladder.

These symptoms are known as prostatism. Without treatment the obstruction can become so severe as to prevent the bladder emptying at all. If this happens suddenly, it is known as acute retention. It is very obvious and painful and requires immediate treatment. If it happens gradually, a little urine being passed from time to time, then it is called chronic retention. The main problem here is that it may not be noticed for a long time. The bladder wall becomes thickened with the increased pressure and the ureters are compressed where they enter the bladder. The resulting back pressure on the kidneys may damage them. In all these situations, infection of the urine in the bladder (cystitis) is common.

What to do

Prevention. There is no way of preventing enlargement of the prostate from developing. Once there are symptoms of prostatism, investigations should be carried out to check whether the bladder is emptying fully or whether there is residual urine left in the bladder after micturition. If there is residual urine, an operation should be carried out to relieve the obstruction. This prevents the complications of retention and renal damage. Any man with symptoms of prostatism should try to empty his bladder regularly and avoid postponing micturition for long after he first feels the urge to go as this may lead to acute retention.

Treatment, after appropriate investigations, is by operation to remove the part of the gland causing the obstruction. No attempt is made to remove the whole of it.

It is widely thought that a man is unable to lead a normal sex life after a prostate operation and indeed many men do develop some transitory sexual difficulty. However, with patience and good-humoured help from a loving partner, this usually resolves itself. It is important that the couple are prepared for a few failures of erection at first and are not deterred from further attempts.

Cancer of the prostate

If the prostate glands of men who have died of other causes are carefully examined, small latent cancers can be found in 14% of men aged 50 years. The incidence increases with age until it reaches 80% in men over 80. However, most of these never extend beyond the gland itself and even in those that do, it is a very slowly progressing disease. It is therefore a rare cause of death or even of symptoms. Some men with cancer of the prostate live to a ripe old age and die of some other cause long before it shows itself.

Kidney stones

Stones (calculi) develop as small crystals, usually of calcium salts, when the urine is supersaturated. They form in the renal pelvis and may stay there, or pass down the ureter to the bladder. If a stone stays in the kidney it may enlarge and cause damage by pressure, obstruction of flow of urine or by facilitating infection. If it passes into the ureter, it causes trouble only if it gets stuck on the way. If this happens, the ureter is blocked and there is intense pain. If it does not pass, the kidney may be damaged by back pressure from the obstruction. If the stone reaches the bladder, it is usually quickly passed to the outside. In the past, it was common for stones to stay in the bladder and increase in size, causing severe pain. One of the earliest operations ever performed was 'cutting for stone'. This was for stones in the bladder and is referred to by Hippocrates. The reasons for the decline in incidence of bladder stones are obscure.

Nowadays, the commonest problem is of ureteric calculus, i.e. a stone stuck in a ureter. A stone need not be more than a millimetre across to cause problems.

What are the effects?

The main symptom is of pain, known as ureteric colic. It is severe and comes and goes in waves (i.e. colic). It starts in the renal angle (loin) of the affected side and moves downwards along the line of the ureter as the stone moves (see Figure 20.3). Typically it goes into the groin or scrotum.

In most cases, the stone passes naturally and all that is needed is plentiful fluids and pain relief. If it fails to pass, it can be removed through a cystoscope.

Prevention

Some people seem to be more likely to develop stones than others and they are particularly likely to develop in someone who is dehydrated (i.e. short of fluid) and producing highly concentrated urine. The most important preventative measure is therefore a high fluid intake, especially in hot weather or during intense exercise.

21

Cancer

What is it?

Cancer is no single disease. It is a general disease process, just as inflammation or healing. Each organ affected will produce its own set of features that patient and doctor can feel and detect. Each cancer will require its own form of treatment. Each has its own favourable or unfavourable outlook.

The term 'cancer' refers to a process whereby certain cells within an organ start to grow independently. The growth is disordered and uncontrolled. Cancer cells have the ability to invade and destroy adjacent structures. They also have the ability to spread to other parts of the body and set up their invasive growth processes there.

Cancer cells grow at variable rates. Some take years to make themselves known, such as cancers of the uterine cervix. Others, such as some cancers of the breast, can be seen to progress and grow quickly.

Cancer is largely a disease of ageing and most cancers affect persons in their later stages of life. However, some — such as leukaemias, Hodgkin's disease, and some bone cancers — tend to affect children.

Cancer is frightening and frightful but it is a relatively uncommon disease and now the outlook with some cancers is good.

Who gets it?

Out of 60 million deaths yearly in the world, only 5 million are caused by cancers — most are caused by infections and malnutrition in young children and infants in developing countries.

In a developed country such as the UK or USA about one quarter of all deaths are caused by cancers.

To get a more local viewpoint, a family physician caring for the average number of 2500 persons can expect to diagnose no more than 7—8 new cancers in a year (see Table 21.1).

Table 21.1   Occurrence of cancer in a general practice of 2500 patients

Type of cancer	No. of cases	Time
Lung	1—2	Yearly
Breast	1	Yearly
Bowel	1	Yearly
Skin	1	Yearly
Stomach	2	3 yearly
Cervix	1	3 yearly
Leukaemia	1	5 yearly
Ovary	1	6 yearly

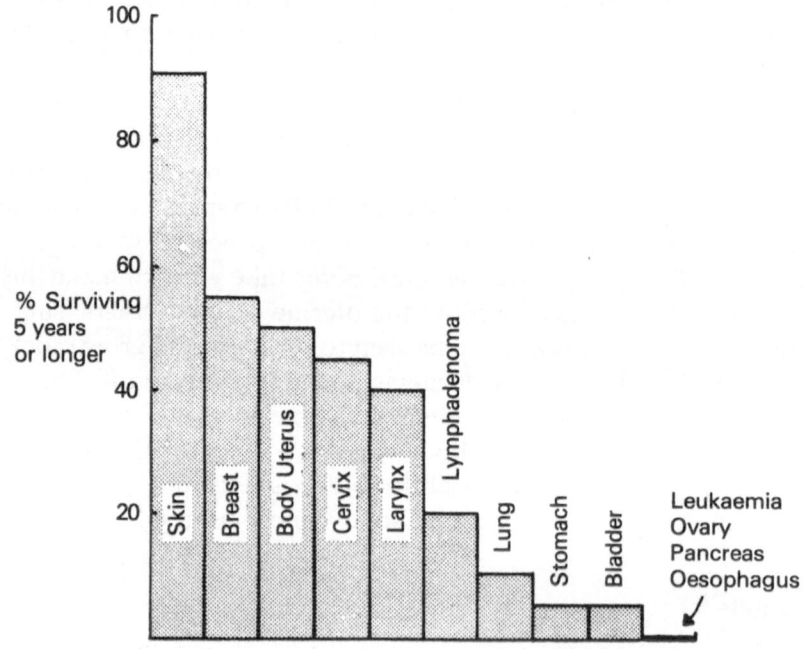

Figure 21.1   Cancer — outlook for cure.

What happens?

Although cancer can be a fatal disease and many do cause death there are many that can be cured or controlled. Figure 21.1 shows the proportions of my patients with certain cancers who have been apparently cured of cancer.

Note the good outlook with skin cancer and the fair outlook with breast, womb (uterus), and laryngeal cancers. The outlook for cancers of the lung, stomach, and leukaemia is poor.

How do they present?

Since each cancer varies and has its own characteristic features the presentation may be different. The following are general comments.

Any change from the normal working or function of a system for more than a week or two should be noted and if it persists warrants assessment by a doctor. Thus, unusual indigestion, a persistent cough, headache and vomiting, or changed bowel habits may be warning features.

Locally, the cancer may present as a *lump* in a breast or on the skin. It may present as enlarged glands in the neck, groin, or elsewhere.

The surface of the growing tumour may become ulcerated and cause abnormal *bleeding*. This may manifest itself as blood-stained sputum, or as passage of blood from the rectum or vagina, or in urine.

There are many other possible presentations such as:

General debility, weakness, loss of weight, and anaemia.
Abdominal swelling.
Persistent pain in chest, abdomen, back, or elsewhere.
Jaundice, fits, loss of voice, and others.

What to do

The earlier the diagnosis of cancer is made the better the chance of cure. Therefore, the role of the individual must be to take to his or her normal physician any unusual, abnormal symptoms that may be lasting and causing problems. They may appear unimportant, but it is the role of the physician to make an assessment and to decide if any further investigations are required — or whether he or she can offer reassurance that the symptoms are unimportant.

Since early diagnosis is important it is reasonable to expect that *screening for cancer by a regular medical check-up* would be helpful.

Unfortunately, there is little evidence that such medical check-ups improve the outlook for cancer patients.

It is much more important that the patient should be observant, sensitive, and intelligent enough to take note of possible early symptoms and seek early advice and help of his or her physician.

Until a reliable blood, or other, screening test for hidden early cancer is available medical check-up screening tests are at best crude and unreliable.

Curative treatment

The current treatments that are available for treating cancer are based on removal or destruction of the growth and preventing recurrence.

The destruction can be achieved by:

Removal of the growth, hopefully completely.
Killing the cancer cells by radiotherapy.
Killing the cancer cells by cytotoxic (cell-destroying) drugs.
Other special measures designed specifically for particular growths.

Prevention

At present the best hope for cancer control is in *prevention* and much of this lies in our own hands.

The best hope for control lies in avoiding environmental irritants that may act as causes of some cancers. The best example on which to take action now is cancer of the lung, which is definitely related to cigarette smoking. Not smoking is the best form of preventing cancer of the lung.

Other possibilities for prevention are in occupational hazards from dusts, fumes, and chemicals; but this requires much more work.

Appendix 1:

How to stop smoking

Your physical and psychological addiction to tobacco can only be overcome by willpower and determination. Unless you really want to stop you will not be able to. There is no point in trying to cut down gradually — you must stop smoking completely from NOW.

Within days of stopping you will notice improved senses of taste and smell, less morning cough and wheeze and less shortness of breath on exercising. In time you may well notice that colds and coughs do not affect either you or your children as often or as severely as before. Remember children of non-smokers are less likely to start smoking themselves.

Most important of all your chances of developing a serious smoking-induced disease (e.g. cancer of the lung, heart attack) are reduced and continue to decrease every day you don't smoke. It is never too late to benefit from stopping, so:

A. Stop now.

B. Throw away your cigarettes, matches, lighters, ashtrays, etc.

C. Never have 'just' one more cigarette.

D. Try to get your family to stop with you and to give you help and encouragement.

E. Tell everyone you know you have stopped so they will not offer you cigarettes and will help maintain your willpower.

F.   Avoid places where people smoke and situations where you used to enjoy smoking most, at least until you are confident you have well and truly beaten the habit.

G.   Every day save the money you would have spent on cigarettes and use it to reward yourself by buying some luxury you could not otherwise have afforded.

There are many aids to help you stop smoking including hypnotism, special filter cigarette holders, nicotine chewing gum and acupuncture. All may help individual smokers to give up but none are a substitute for willpower and determination.

Appendix 2:

Fast diet

The diet is for two weeks only; do not substitute items.

Abstain from everything not included in the diet and be sure to eat only what is assigned rather than do without.

No eating between meals; take all vegetables without butter; all salads without oil; use lean parts of meat. Coffee must be black, and tea clear. Water — no restriction of amount drunk. Eggs must be boiled or poached but not scrambled or fried.

Breakfast

The same every morning: grapefruit, one or two eggs, and coffee or tea.

Monday

Lunch: Two eggs, tomato, and coffee.
Dinner: Two eggs, combination salad, one piece of toast (dry), grapefruit, and coffee.

Tuesday

Lunch: Two eggs, tomato, and coffee.
Dinner: Steak, tomatoes, cucumber, lettuce, olives, and coffee.

Wednesday

Lunch: Two eggs, spinach, and coffee.
Dinner: Two lamb chops, celery, cucumber, tomatoes, and tea.

Thursday

Lunch: Two eggs, spinach, and coffee.
Dinner: Two eggs, cottage cheese, cabbage, and one piece of toast (dry).

Friday

Lunch: Two eggs, spinach, and coffee.
Dinner: Fish, combination salad, dry toast, and grapefruit.

Saturday

Lunch: Fruit salad; put in everything, as much as you want.
Dinner: Plenty of steak, celery, cucumber, tomatoes, and coffee.

Sunday

Lunch: Cold chicken, tomatoes, and grapefruit.
Dinner: Chicken, tomatoes, carrots, cabbage, grapefruit, and coffee.

Warning: *Do not stay on this diet for more than two weeks.*

Body weight should drop about 6.4—9.5 kg (14—20 lb) in two weeks; the basis of the diet is chemical. The quantity consumed is not important, except where stated. Scotch may be consumed in moderate amounts on days when meat is eaten; for a prodigious drinker, this would be about three drinks with water. Carbonated drinks must not be taken, unless of the one-calorie variety.

Appendix 3:

Diet for healthy living

(1) Change to wholemeal bread and eat at least five to six slices every day. You can easily manage this amount if you have sandwiches or toast for two meals each day. If you cannot obtain wholemeal then eat Granary or wheatgerm — even brown bread is better than white! The fattening power of sandwiches comes not from the bread but from what you put between the slices!

(2) Start the day with breakfast — either cereal or toast with egg or bacon, etc. If you cannot take breakfast, take wholemeal bread sandwiches to eat during the morning.

(3) Eat more potatoes, vegetables, and fruit. Aim to double the amount you have at present and choose a dark green vegetable or carrots at least three times a week.

(4) Have only a thin spread of butter or margarine on bread, or change to a low-fat spread like Gold or Outline. Soft and ordinary margarines are fattening as butter. If you find that sandwiches are too dry, fill them with moist foods like pickle, tomato, lettuce, cress, grated carrot, raw cabbage, chutney, banana, or jam.

(5) Eat less fried food, cakes, gateaux, pastry, biscuits, and puddings. Try halving the amount you have at first, and aim to have no more than one of each every week. Fill up on bread and choose bread rather than chips if there are no boiled, baked, or mashed potatoes on the menu.

(6) Always cut the fat off meat. Cut down on fatty foods in recipes (like butter, margarine, cream, and oil). There is no need to fry meat or mince before stewing or casseroling it; use gravy powder or browning for colour.

(7) Cheese, eggs, and most meat (even lean meat) are high in fat so eat less of these. It does not matter if you do not eat meat every day. The exceptions are chicken, turkey, rabbit, liver, kidney, and white fish, which are low in fat — but do not fry them.

(8) Choose silver or red-top milk, not gold top. Use plain yoghurt instead of cream where possible, and try using dried skimmed milk for sauces and milk puddings. (Some products may have skimmed milk with added vegetable fats — avoid these.)

(9) Give up sugar in tea and coffee by reducing the amount used then giving it up completely. This is better than keeping your 'sweet tooth' by using saccharin. Having given up sugar most people then dislike sweet drinks. Eat fruit instead of sweets and puddings.

(10) Soft drinks are fattening unless they state that they have only one calorie per ounce per bottle. 'Diabetic lager' is just as fattening as ordinary lager. Choose a low-calorie drink or plain water.

Index